THE 30-DA`

FOOD COOKBOOK FOR

BEGINNERS

Revitalize Your Life in Just One Month with Simple, Tasty Whole
Food Recipes to Jumpstart Your Health Without the Hassle

Nancy Walton

TABLE OF CONTENTS

CHAPTER 13: MAINTAINING A WHOLE FOOD LIFESTYLE 103

CHAPTER 1: WHOLE FOOD ESSENTIALS

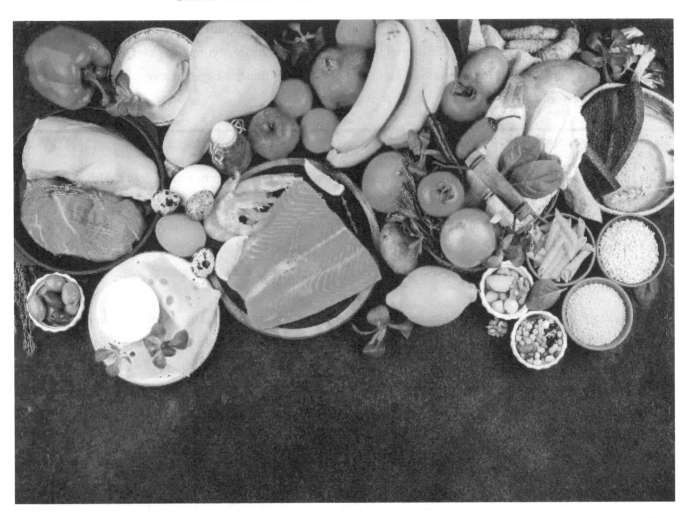

Welcome to your first steps on a transformative journey with whole foods—a path that's not only about nourishing your body but revitalizing your entire life. The essence of whole foods lies in their simplicity and integrity; these are the foods that come to us without heavy processing, retaining their full nutritional profiles and natural flavors.

Imagine this: you're at the local farmer's market, standing amid vibrant stands bursting with fresh produce. Here, every season is marked by its offerings—crisp apples in fall, succulent strawberries in spring. These whole foods are as close to nature as they can get, and starting your journey here means beginning a dialogue with your food that asks, "What goodness will you bring me?"

There's a compelling reason why a whole food diet is so lauded: the benefits are manifold. From enhancing digestion—imagine saying goodbye to those pesky bouts of bloat and discomfort—to elevating your energy levels so significantly that you may discover reservoirs of vigor you never knew you had. Moreover, it's not merely about physical wellness; the mental clarity that comes from a clean, wholesome diet can often feel like fog lifting from your mind.

Yet, embarking on this path isn't without its hurdles. Change always requires a level of adaptation, and the shift to whole foods is no different. Whether you're concerned about the time it may take to prepare whole food meals amid a busy lifestyle, or wondering how you'll coax your family into enjoying heartier grains and less sugar, these initial steps are about setting the groundwork. It involves cultivating a mindset that views these changes as exciting opportunities rather than cumbersome challenges.

So, within these pages, we delve deep into what constitutes whole foods, uncover their profound impact on health, and lay out practical, manageable strategies to integrate them into your life. You're embarking on a journey that promises to be as delicious as it is nourishing. Consider this the beginning of a beautiful friendship between you and whole foods—one that's built to last a lifetime.

• 1.1 UNDERSTANDING WHOLE FOODS

Whole foods are often spoken of in a mystical sense, as if merely uttering the term can bestow health and vitality. But beyond the buzz, what really defines these ingredients? Quite simply, they are foods that have been processed or refined as little as possible and are free from additives or other artificial substances. Picture an apple freshly plucked from a tree, a handful of unadulterated almonds, or a fillet of salmon caught in the wild— these are more than just parts of a meal; they are whole foods, complete with their natural nutrients and inherent benefits.

Understanding whole foods is akin to relearning how to eat as nature intended. Historically, our ancestors' diets were not made up of the pre-packaged, sugar-laden, or deep-fried items commonly available today. They ate what the land provided—seasonal fruits and veggies, grains, legumes, meats, and fish. This natural diet provided them with all the necessary nutrients to live, work, and thrive. In many ways, shifting our diet back to this natural state is a nod to a time when eating was simpler and, quite likely, healthier.

The Richness of Nutrients

Whole foods are powerhouses of essential nutrients. These foods are rich in vitamins, minerals, dietary fiber, and antioxidants, while remaining low on additives and artificial ingredients that might detract from their beneficial properties. For example, consider the difference between an orange and a bottle of processed orange juice. The former contains fibers, full vitamin content, and natural sugars, as processed in your body more slowly than the often sugar-enhanced juice counterpart.

The fiber in whole foods, such as fruits, vegetables, and whole grains, supports digestive health by helping to maintain bowel regularity and by stabilizing glucose levels. The vitamins and minerals found in these unprocessed foods are crucial for bodily functions such as energy production, immune defense, and cell repair.

The Hidden Perils of Processed Foods

To truly appreciate the value of whole foods, it's essential to recognize what they are not. They are the antithesis of processed foods, which are often stripped of nutrients and laden with unhealthy additives like excess sodium, sugars, and trans fats. Frequent consumption of heavily processed foods has been linked to various health issues, including elevated risks of obesity, heart disease, high blood pressure, and diabetes. The contrast between the potential health risks associated with a diet rich in processed foods and the benefits of a whole foods-based diet couldn't be starker.

Whole Foods and Energy Levels

Switching to a whole food diet may also have an impressive effect on your energy levels. The slow and steady digestion of these natural foods provides a constant source of energy, as opposed to the rapid spikes and subsequent crashes caused by high-sugar or high-fat processed foods. Many people who embrace whole foods report enhanced overall vitality, better focus, and improved mood—all of which can be attributed to better blood sugar balance and the body receiving the nutrients it needs to perform at its best.

Sustainable and Ethical Eating

Moreover, a shift towards whole foods is a shift towards more sustainable eating habits. Local fruits and vegetables, seasonal produce, and grass-fed as well as free-range meats are generally considered more environmentally friendly than mass-produced processed items. This is due to less energy spent on processing, packaging, and transporting these foods. By choosing whole foods, you're not only making a decision that benefits your health but also one that contributes less to environmental degradation.

Integrating Whole Foods into Your Diet

The journey to integrating more whole foods into your diet is both a mental and physical transition. It starts with a decision to prioritize your health and a willingness to explore a variety of foods perhaps previously overlooked. It doesn't mean you need to overhaul your entire pantry overnight or never again indulge in a favorite treat. Rather, it's about making a conscious effort to choose more natural, less processed items as the staples of your diet.

Whether it's replacing breakfast cereals with oats topped with fresh berries, choosing whole grain over white bread, or preparing a home-cooked meal with fresh ingredients instead of opening a can, these small changes can collectively lead to substantial health improvements. Each meal presents an opportunity to make choices that align more closely with a whole food-based diet.

Rediscovering the Joy of Eating

Part of embracing whole foods is rediscovering the flavors and textures that might have been masked by processing. It's about learning to appreciate the crispness of a fresh salad, the robustness of whole grain bread, or the natural sweetness of ripe fruit. This re-education of the palate can open up a new world of culinary experiences and appreciation for simple, nourishing meals.

Whole foods bring us back to the basics of eating — to choices that enrich our bodies and minds. By understanding the intrinsic value of these foods, acknowledging their myriad benefits, and deciding to integrate them more fully into our daily lives, we commit to a sustainable, healthful lifestyle that honors our bodies and the environment. Embracing whole foods is not just a diet trend; it's a lasting approach to eating that celebrates natural nutrition, simplicity, and life-enhancing wholesomeness. So, let the journey begin with understanding, continue with integration, and thrive on the rejuvenation that whole foods can bring into your life.

• 1.2 THE HEALTH IMPACTS

Embarking on a whole food diet is like setting forth on a gentle yet profound revolution within your body. The immediate benefits on your digestion and energy levels are just the tip of the iceberg. Over time, this foundation paves the way for long-term wellness, affecting every part of your being from your morning vitality to your nighttime rest.

Improving Digestive Health

Starting with the very core of our well-being, digestion, whole foods offer unparalleled benefits. High in fiber and free from disruptive additives, these foods help maintain a healthy gut flora, which is crucial for efficient digestion. Fiber plays a pivotal role here; it's not only essential for regular bowel movements but also feeds the beneficial bacteria in our gut. This beneficial bacteria helps combat inflammation and produce vital nutrients such as vitamins B and K.

Imagine your digestive system as a well-tuned orchestra where each instrument plays its part in harmony. Whole foods provide the sheet music for this orchestra, guiding each component to perform optimally. Processed foods, however, can be likened to a cacophony disrupting this harmony. They might provide temporary pleasure but confuse the delicate balance of our digestive processes.

Boosting Energy Levels

On the energy front, whole foods are akin to a slow-burning fuel that powers us throughout the day. Unlike the fleeting surge of energy we get from sugar-laden snacks, the complex carbohydrates in whole foods provide a steady release. This means no drastic spikes and troughs in blood sugar levels, just a consistent supply of vitality. Consider a day powered by whole foods: starting with a breakfast of oatmeal topped with fresh berries, a midday meal of quinoa salad loaded with veggies, and a dinner featuring grilled salmon and steamed greens. Each meal is designed to sustain and nourish without leaving you fatigued after eating.

Promoting Long-Term Wellness

The long-term health impacts of a whole food diet can be profound. Regular consumption of fruits, vegetables, lean proteins, and whole grains has been shown to reduce the risk of major lifestyle diseases such as heart disease, diabetes, and obesity. These foods are dense in antioxidants, which fight against oxidative stress—a culprit in aging and many chronic diseases. Additionally, the anti-inflammatory properties of many whole foods can alleviate chronic inflammation, a persistent state of distress in the body linked to numerous health issues.

Chronic inflammation is an insidious enemy, often lurking without loud symptoms until significant damage is done. Incorporating anti-inflammatory foods into your diet acts like soothing balm, gradually reducing this silent inflammation and restoring your body's equilibrium.

Enhancing Mental Health and Mood

The benefits of a whole food diet extend beyond the physical. There's a compelling link between diet and mental health, often referred to as the gut-brain axis. Our gut microbiota plays a vital role in producing and regulating neurotransmitters like serotonin, which predominantly resides in our gut. A diet rich in whole foods supports the health of our gut microbiota, subsequently enhancing our mood and cognitive function.

The mental clarity that emerges from a whole food diet can feel like lifting a fog you didn't know was there. Imagine improved focus, better memory retention, and a more stable mood—all facilitated by the simple choice of what you put on your plate.

Aiding Weight Management

Furthermore, for those concerned with maintaining a healthy weight, a whole food diet offers a sustainable and effective solution. These foods are typically less calorie-dense yet more filling due to their high fiber content. This makes it easier to satisfy hunger with fewer calories, naturally supporting weight management without the need for restrictive dieting.

The journey of eating whole foods is one of reconnection with your body's natural signals—recognizing true hunger and feeling genuinely satiated. It dismantles the cycle of cravings and guilt associated with diets heavy in processed foods, establishing a healthier relationship with food.

Cultivating Radiant Skin

Lastly, the external benefits shouldn't be overlooked. Healthy eating reflects on the outside, too. Nutrients in whole foods such as vitamins A, C, and E, as well as omega-3 fatty acids, play a crucial role in skin health. They help protect the skin from oxidative damage that can lead to premature aging, and aid in keeping the skin hydrated and resilient.

A whole food diet might then be visualized as a fountain of youth, sustaining your body's health from the inside out, and reflecting that vitality through clear, glowing skin.

In summary, transitioning to a whole food diet isn't just a dietary change—it's a lifestyle overhaul that bolsters your digestion, energizes your days, and fortifies your long-term health. Each meal becomes an opportunity not just to satisfy taste buds, but to heal, energize, and renew your body. It's about building a foundation of well-being that supports not only yourself but also nurtures the planet. Therefore, whole foods offer more than just sustenance; they are a recipe for a vibrant, healthier life.

• 1.3 PREPARING FOR CHANGE

Embarking on a journey to embrace whole foods in your diet is much like preparing for a voyage. It requires planning, preparation, and most importantly, a shift in your mindset. Your readiness to change not only impacts your initial steps but also determines how effectively you maintain this healthier way of eating in the long run.

Crafting Your Whole Foods Mindset

The first step in your journey is not to stock up your pantry (yet!), but to cultivate the right mindset. Shift your perspective from seeing this change as depriving yourself of certain foods, to nourishing your body with others. This positive mindset focuses on abundance rather than restriction, which can make the transition smoother and more enjoyable.

Consider why you are making this change. Is it for better health? More energy? To support a sustainable planet? Keep these reasons clear in your mind, as they will motivate you when challenges arise. Setting intentions is like setting your coordinates on a map; they guide your journey and keep you moving in the right direction.

Informing Yourself and Setting Goals

Once your mindset aligns with your new dietary aspirations, the next step is education. Understanding the principles of whole foods and their benefits arms you with valuable knowledge that can inspire and guide your choices. Read books, watch documentaries, or even attend workshops to immerse yourself in the whole food philosophy. This groundwork not only solidifies your commitment but also makes you more adept at making healthy choices instinctively.

With knowledge in hand, it's time to set practical, achievable goals. Maybe your initial goal is to incorporate a whole food-based meal into your diet once a day or to eliminate processed sugars progressively. These goals should be specific, measurable, achievable, relevant, and time-bound (SMART). By setting such targets, you create a framework that can foster success and allow you to track your progress effectively.

Preparing Your Environment

The environment around you can significantly influence your eating habits. Start by making your kitchen a sanctuary for whole foods. Clear out heavily processed foods from your pantry and refrigerator. Stock up on whole grains, legumes, nuts, seeds, and fresh produce. When whole foods are the easiest option available, you're more likely to choose them.

Consider where you shop as well. Local farmers' markets and health food stores often carry a wider range of fresh, whole food options than conventional supermarkets. Plus, the food from these sources is typically less processed, and buying local supports sustainable agriculture—a win for your health and the planet.

Incorporating Whole Foods Gradually

While some may prefer an immediate and total shift, for many, a gradual transition to whole foods is more sustainable. Start by introducing whole food versions of foods you already enjoy. Love pasta? Try whole grain or legume-based options. Adore sweets? Opt for natural sources like fruits or honey. Over time, your palate will start to appreciate and crave the natural flavors of whole foods.

Tracking Progress and Adjusting Habits

Monitoring your progress is crucial as it keeps you motivated and helps identify areas that need adjustment. Keep a food diary or use a mobile app to track what you eat, how much, and how it makes you feel. This record can be incredibly eye-opening, allowing you to make correlations between your diet and energy levels, digestion, and overall wellness.

As you progress, adjust your goals and methods if necessary. If you find that a certain approach isn't working, tweak it until you find a rhythm that suits you. Flexibility in your approach can prevent frustration and ensure that your transition to whole foods remains enjoyable rather than becoming a chore.

Building a Support System

Change can be challenging, so it's important to surround yourself with support. Share your goals with friends or family members who might also be interested in improving their diet. Alternatively, join online communities where you can find encouragement and share experiences with like-minded individuals. Sometimes, the journey is easier when you know you're not navigating it alone.

Celebrating Wins and Refining Your Journey

Every step towards a whole food lifestyle is a victory that should be celebrated. Acknowledge your efforts, whether it's resisting the temptation of processed snacks or successfully preparing a whole food feast for your family. These positive affirmations can reinforce your commitment and boost your morale.

As you settle into your whole foods journey, continue to refine your approach. Learn from each experience, and don't hesitate to expand your palate and try new, exciting foods. Whole food eating is not just about health; it's about discovering a world of flavors and enjoying food in its most natural and nutritious form.

In essence, preparing for a diet rich in whole foods is a comprehensive process that extends far beyond mere food choices. It involves a deep-seated commitment to better living—a decision to nourish your body and mind with the best nature has to offer. With the right mindset, knowledge, and support, the shift to whole foods can not only be successful but also deeply fulfilling.

CHAPTER 2: 30-DAY WHOLE FOOD CHALLENGE

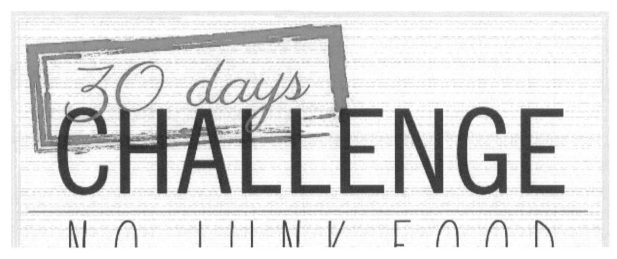

Embarking on a 30-day whole food challenge is like standing at the threshold of a new home; you're ready to open the door to a life brimming with vitality, clarity, and joy. As you read these lines, envision yourself harnessing the earth's bounty, transforming simple ingredients into meals that nourish and revitalize. This journey is not just about eating differently; it's about redefining your relationship with food.

Imagine a pantry where every item is chosen with intention, free from preservatives and artificial additives. These are the foundations of whole foods—foods that are minimally processed, rich in nutrients, and inherently satisfying. Over the next 30 days, as you progressively fill your kitchen and your plate with these wholesome selections, you'll likely notice subtle yet profound changes. Your morning fatigue might dwindle, replaced by a surge of energy that doesn't fade with the setting sun. That afternoon slump that once had you reaching for a sugary pick-me-up? It might just become a part of your past.

But let's be clear, the path to transformative change is not always lined with ease. The commitment to prepare and cook fresh, whole foods daily requires both time and creativity. However, think of this not as a challenge, but as an exploration—an adventure where each meal is an opportunity to discover new flavors and textures. As with any expedition, preparation is key. Setting up your kitchen with essential tools and staple ingredients, understanding effective meal planning, and learning efficient shopping strategies will equip you to face this challenge head-on.

By embracing this 30-day whole food challenge, you're not just feeding your body; you're nurturing your soul. You'll learn to appreciate the natural tastes of food, to enjoy the process of cooking, and to take pride in the meals you've created. This chapter is designed to guide, inspire, and prepare you for this transformative journey—a journey that starts with simple decisions in the kitchen and leads to lasting changes in the way you feel, think, and live. So, tie on your apron and let's begin this fulfilling expedition together.

• 2.1 PANTRY PREPARATION

Stepping into your kitchen to embark on the 30-day whole food challenge, the heart of your culinary domain becomes the pantry—a veritable treasure chest that, when properly stocked, can transform the ordinary into the sublime. Properly preparing this space is like drawing the map for a journey; it outlines the route, ensures all necessary provisions are on hand, and ensures every meal is a step towards renewed health and vitality.

Creating a Whole Food Pantry Sanctuary

When you first open your pantry door, what greets you? Are the shelves cluttered with cans of unknown origin, half-empty boxes of processed snacks, and jumbled spices from years ago? Let the first step towards your whole food transformation be clearing out the non-essentials. This doesn't mean waste—consider donating unopened, non-perishable items that aren't part of your whole food plan or finding inventive ways to incorporate them into last pre-challenge meals.

With space cleared, your pantry is now a blank canvas, ready to be stocked with the vibrant colors of whole food ingredients. Think of your pantry as a garden; everything you place here will eventually flourish into your meals, so choose wisely and with purpose.

The Staples of Whole Food Cooking

Grains and Legumes

Whole grains and legumes are the cornerstone of many healthy dishes, offering essential proteins, fiber, and B vitamins. Stocking up on varieties like quinoa, brown rice, and oats ensures that you have a ready base for meals. Also, consider lentils, chickpeas, and various beans, which can be cooked in bulk and stored for convenience. Opt for dry over canned to reduce exposure to sodium and preservatives.

Nuts and Seeds

A small handful of unsalted almonds, walnuts, or cashews not only makes an excellent snack but can also transform a salad, yogurt, or breakfast bowl into a satisfying meal with a crunch. Similarly, seeds such as chia, flax, and pumpkin seeds are tiny nutrition powerhouses rich in omega-3 fatty acids and fiber. Store these in airtight containers to maintain freshness and sprinkle liberally to add texture and nutrients to your dishes.

Oils and Vinegars

The right oils and vinegars can elevate a dish from ordinary to extraordinary. Stock your pantry with quality olive oil for cooking and salad dressings, coconut oil for its high heat tolerance and sweet aroma, and perhaps walnut or avocado oil for their unique flavors. Acidity from vinegars like apple cider, red wine, and balsamic can not only flavor salads but can also balance and brighten heavier dishes.

Herbs and Spices

Fresh herbs may come and go with the seasons, but a well-stocked spice cupboard will always provide the backbone for flavor in your cooking. Basics like black pepper, basil, oregano, and cinnamon are a must, but also explore turmeric, cumin, coriander, and ginger to add depth and unique twists to your meals. Always aim for whole spices as they retain their potency longer and can be ground when needed.

Sweeteners

While reducing refined sugar is a pillar of the whole food diet, having natural sweeteners on hand for occasional use can aid the transition. Raw honey, pure maple syrup, and dates are excellent choices for adding a touch of sweetness to recipes without spiking your blood sugar levels like processed sugars would.

The Art of Smart Shopping

With a clear idea of what your pantry will hold, shopping becomes less of a chore and more of an extension of your whole food philosophy. Here are tips to keep you focused and efficient on your shopping trips:

- **Prioritize Whole Foods**: Always navigate to the perimeter of the grocery store first. This is typically where the unprocessed foods are found—fresh fruits, vegetables, meats, and dairy products. The aisles should be your last stop for whole grains, nuts, and seeds, ensuring you don't fall into the processed foods trap.

- **Read Labels**: Even on the outskirts of the store, it's crucial to read labels. Look for products with ingredients you recognize and can pronounce. The fewer the ingredients, the closer the food is to its natural state.
- **Buy in Bulk**: Many whole food staples like grains and legumes are available in bulk, which can save money and reduce packaging waste. Only buy what you can realistically use before it spoils to avoid wastage.
- **Seasonal and Local**: Whenever possible, choose seasonal and local produce. These options are generally fresher and more flavorful, making them a joy to cook with. Plus, supporting local farmers helps sustain your community's economy and reduces the environmental impact of long-distance food transport.

Embracing the Whole Food Pantry

As your challenge progresses, you'll find that a well-organized, thoughtfully stocked pantry isn't just a tool for health—it's a cornerstone of your lifestyle change. Your pantry becomes a gateway to nourishing meals that not only feed your body but also bring delight and satisfaction in their creation. With each spice, each grain, each carefully selected oil, you're crafting a foundation for lasting health, and more importantly, a passion for wholesome, vibrant cooking that can last a lifetime. This is the true essence of the whole food challenge—a journey that goes far beyond mere diet and into the heart of a joyfully sustainable way of living.

• 2.2 ESSENTIAL TOOLS

As you embark on the 30-Day Whole Food Challenge, your kitchen becomes your laboratory, and just as any skilled scientist needs the right equipment, so too do you need the proper tools to transform raw ingredients into nourishing meals. Equipping your kitchen with essential tools not only simplifies your meal preparation but also enhances your cooking experience, making it seamless and more enjoyable.

Imagine your kitchen as a workshop where each tool has a specific role in creating your culinary masterpieces. The right set of tools can be the difference between a meal that is simply functional and one that is truly delightful.

THE FOUNDATION OF EVERY GREAT KITCHEN

High-Quality Knives

A chef's knife and a paring knife are indispensable in any kitchen. These knives should be made of high-carbon steel for durability and precision. A sharp chef's knife, typically 8 inches long, effortlessly chops vegetables, slices meat, and minces herbs. In contrast, a smaller paring knife is perfect for peeling and trimming. Investing in good knives, and keeping them sharp, not only makes prepping ingredients faster but also safer.

Cutting Boards

Consider pairing your knives with a selection of cutting boards. Having multiple boards prevents cross-contamination between produce and proteins. Opt for bamboo or thick plastic boards that are easy on knife blades and dishwasher safe for convenient cleaning.

THE MECHANICS OF COOKING

High-Performance Blender

A robust blender opens up a world of possibility for soups, smoothies, dressings, and even whole-food juices. High-speed blenders can pulverize nuts into butter, transform dates into puree, and crush ice into the snow, making them a versatile tool in a whole food kitchen.

Food Processor

Similar to the blender, but distinct in its capabilities, a food processor is ideal for slicing vegetables, grinding nuts and seeds, making dough, and combining ingredients for patties or meatballs. It is particularly useful for batch cooking as it reduces preparation time significantly.

Sturdy Pots and Pans

A set of stainless steel and/or cast-iron cookware is essential for even heat distribution and non-reactive cooking. A good sauté pan, a large stockpot, and a heavy-bottom skillet cover most cooking needs from sautéing vegetables to simmering hearty stews.

SUPPORTING ACTS

Measuring Cups and Spoons

Accuracy is key in creating dishes that taste consistently good. Measuring cups and spoons ensure that you add ingredients in proportions that are tried and tested. They are particularly handy when experimenting with new recipes or baking, where precision is crucial.

Mixing Bowls

A nesting set of mixing bowls in various sizes makes meal preparation orderly and efficient. Whether you are tossing a salad or marinating protein, having a range of sizes ensures you have the right bowl for the task at hand.

Grater and Vegetable Peeler

These tools might seem simple, but they are time savers. A sharp vegetable peeler can make quick work of carrots, cucumbers, and potatoes, while a four-sided grater offers options for coarse or fine grating of cheese and vegetables.

SPECIAL MENTIONS

Instant Pot or Slow Cooker

These appliances deserve a special mention for their convenience and versatility. An Instant Pot, which combines several kitchen appliances in one (pressure cooker, slow cooker, rice cooker, etc.), is particularly effective for healthy, one-pot meals. A slow cooker is invaluable for those who value coming home to a warm, ready-to-eat dinner after a long day.

Silicone Baking Mats or Parchment Paper

For those who lean towards baking, silicone mats or parchment paper are essential for non-stick baking and easy clean-up, allowing you to forgo adding excessive oil or butter.

Spice Grinder

Finally, a spice grinder unlocks the full potential of spices by allowing you to grind them fresh. Fresh-ground spices maintain more of their essential oils and flavor compared to pre-ground, enhancing the taste and aromatics of your dishes.

Assembling Your Toolkit

Setting up your kitchen with these tools doesn't have to be a daunting expense. Start with the basics and gradually add items that fit your cooking style and needs. Many cooks find joy in the hunt for kitchen tools, whether scouring online deals or exploring local stores for high-quality products.

As you grow into your whole food journey, you'll discover which tools you reach for most often and which you can do without. Each kitchen is as unique as the cook who works in it, and the tools you select become extensions of your culinary ambitions. With a well-set kitchen, every meal becomes an opportunity to explore, experiment, and expand your skills.

Remember, the right tool not only does the job effectively but also adds to the joy of cooking. Whether it's a perfectly balanced knife, a powerful blender, or a dependable pot, each tool in your kitchen contributes to the ease and success of your whole food preparations. Embrace these tools as partners in your culinary adventure on the 30-Day Whole Food Challenge.

• 2.3 PLANNING AND PREP

When beginning your 30-Day Whole Food Challenge, the magic lies in the mastery of meal planning, batch cooking, and savvy shopping strategies. These are not just practices but transformative rituals that will redefine your relationship with food. They are your stepping stones to success, ensuring that each meal supports your health goals and fits seamlessly into your hectic schedule.

The Art of Meal Planning

Starting your journey requires a map, and in the world of whole food cooking, your meal plan is just that. It's a concrete plan for what you will eat over the next week or month. Begin by envisioning your week: meetings, family commitments, evenings out. Each of these affects your meal times and choices.

A well-thought-out meal plan reflects not just your dietary goals but also your real life. On busy days, perhaps a slow cooker stew is perfect, bubbling away while you work, ready when you return. On more flexible days, experimenting with a new recipe might be just the culinary adventure you need.

How do you begin charting this map? Sit down once a week with your favorite recipe sources—perhaps a mix of trusted cookbooks and food blogs—and choose meals that inspire excitement yet call for realistic preparation time considering your schedule. Write down your meal plan, visualizing each meal's place in your week. This plan acts not only as a guide but as a commitment to your health.

Batch Cooking: Your Culinary Time Machine

Imagine cooking portions not just for one meal but for several. This is batch cooking, a method that can significantly lighten your weekly culinary load. It involves preparing large quantities of versatile ingredients or entire meals that are refrigerated or frozen for future use. Think grains, proteins, or a colorful array of roasted vegetables ready to be transformed into quick, nutritious meals.

To effectively batch cook, select one day per week as your cooking day—often a weekend. Cook staples in bulk: grains like quinoa or rice, legumes, and proteins such as chicken or tofu. Simmer a large pot of soup or stew. Roast a variety of vegetables seasoned simply with olive oil, salt, and pepper. Once cooked, store these in the refrigerator or freezer in clearly labeled containers. The beauty of this approach is evident on a hectic weekday evening when a healthy meal is just a matter of reassembly.

Smart Shopping Strategies

Armed with your meal plan, the next step is shopping. This can be a delightful experience if approached with a strategy. Here are a few guidelines to help navigate:

- **Stick to Your List**: Your meal plan translates into a shopping list. Buy what's on the list, nothing more, nothing less. This not only helps manage your budget but also deters impulse buys, which can often be less healthy.

- **Choose Whole and Fresh**: Prioritize fresh fruits and vegetables, whole grains, and fresh meats. When choosing packaged foods, opt for those with minimal and recognizable ingredients.

- **Perimeter Shopping**: Start your shopping trip around the perimeter of the store where fresh produce, dairy, and proteins are often located. Venturing into the aisles might be necessary for staples like spices and oils, but the outer ring is where the majority of whole food shopping is done.

- **Seasonal Selections**: Choose produce that is in season. Not only is it more flavorful and nutrient-dense, but it is also often cheaper and more environmentally friendly.

- **Local and Organic**: When possible, opt for local and organic items. Local products are generally fresher, and organic foods are free from pesticides and genetically modified organisms, aligning closely with whole food principles.

Each of these strategies contributes to a streamlined, stress-free shopping experience, helping you bring home the best ingredients to fuel your challenge.

Integrating Planning, Cooking, and Shopping into Your Routine

To make these practices sustainable, integrate them into your weekly routine. Dedicate specific times for meal planning, shopping, and cooking. Treat these as appointments with yourself, non-negotiable times that are vital for your health. As these become habitual, you'll find they not only become easier but also enjoyable—a time to creatively engage with the food you eat.

Remember, the journey through the Whole Food Challenge is about more than just food; it's about setting a foundation for lasting health and enjoyment in cooking. By mastering meal planning, batch cooking, and smart shopping, you equip yourself with the tools to sustain a healthier lifestyle long after the 30 days are over. These practices are your allies, ensuring that even amidst a busy life, you can maintain a commitment to nourishing yourself and your loved ones with whole, unprocessed, and delightful foods.

CHAPTER 3: BREAKFAST OPTIONS

Morning time—often busy, sometimes chaotic, but always important. It's the moment when the day rolls out before us, ripe with potential and possibility. For many of us, breakfast is a hurried cup of coffee as we dash out the door. Yet, imagine transforming these first crucial moments of your day into a nourishing ritual that sets a tone of health and vitality.

In this chapter on breakfast options, we explore how the simplest meal of the day can also become your most empowering. Whether you're a parent preparing food for an energetic family, or a professional juggling an intense schedule, the recipes shared here are designed to fit seamlessly into your life, imbuing it with wellness and energy.

Think of a breakfast that does more than just fill you up. Envision starting your morning with foods that fuel your body and mind, prepared from wholesome, whole food ingredients that assure both health and satisfaction. We're talking about vibrant smoothie bowls sprinkled with seeds, warm, comforting oats simmered with cinnamon, and light, fluffy pancakes made from almond flour, enjoyed with a swipe of natural peanut butter and a drizzle of raw honey.

Each recipe is crafted to be straightforward and quick, respecting your time constraints while uplifting your health goals. They're dishes that call for minimal prep and can often be made in advance—a perfect match for your fast-paced lifestyle. More so, they're infinitely adaptable, encouraging you to use whatever fresh produce might be available or preferred, fostering a tangible connection between you and your meals.

This is about more than just feeding yourself; it's about setting a foundation for a healthier, more energized life each day. So pour yourself a fresh cup of tea or a smooth, homemade almond milk latte and discover how delightful and vitalizing your mornings can become with just a few tweaks to your breakfast routine.

• 3.1 SMOOTHIES AND SHAKES

GREEN DETOX TWIST

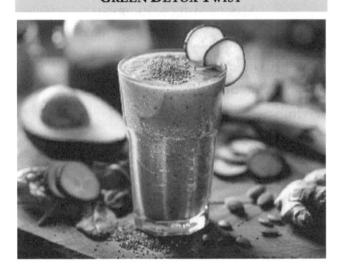

Preparation Time: 10 min.

Cooking Time: none

Mode of Cooking: Blending

Servings: 2

Ingredients:

- 1 cup fresh spinach
- 1 ripe banana
- 1/2 cup cucumber, sliced
- 1/2 avocado
- 1/2-inch piece ginger, peeled
- 1 Tbsp chia seeds
- 2 cups coconut water
- Ice cubes as needed

Directions:

1. Combine spinach, banana, cucumber, avocado, ginger, chia seeds, and coconut water in a blender
2. Blend until smooth and creamy
3. Add ice cubes and blend again until frosty

Tips:

- Add a squeeze of fresh lemon juice for an extra detoxifying effect
- If the smoothie is too thick, adjust the consistency with more coconut water

Nutritional Values: Calories: 180, Fat: 7g, Carbs: 30g, Protein: 3g, Sugar: 12g, Sodium: 110 mg, Potassium: 890 mg, Cholesterol: 0 mg

BERRY IMMUNE BOOSTER

Preparation Time: 10 min.

Cooking Time: none

Mode of Cooking: Blending

Servings: 2

Ingredients:

- 1 cup mixed berries (strawberries, blueberries, raspberries)
- 1 ripe banana
- 1 Tbsp almond butter
- 1 Tbsp flaxseed meal
- 1/2 tsp cinnamon
- 2 cups almond milk
- Ice cubes as needed

Directions:

1. Add all ingredients to a blender
2. Blend until smooth
3. Add ice and blend again to reach desired consistency

Tips:

- Add a scoop of plant-based protein powder for an extra protein boost
- Use frozen berries for a colder and more refreshing smoothie

Nutritional Values: Calories: 230, Fat: 8g, Carbs: 36g, Protein: 5g, Sugar: 20g, Sodium: 180 mg, Potassium: 450 mg, Cholesterol: 0 mg

TROPICAL ENERGY SURGE

Preparation Time: 12 min.

Cooking Time: none

Mode of Cooking: Blending

Servings: 2

Ingredients:

- 1 cup fresh pineapple cubes
- 1 ripe mango, peeled and cubed
- 1/2 cup coconut flakes
- 1 Tbsp hemp seeds
- 1 cup coconut milk
- 1 Tbsp fresh lime juice
- Ice cubes as needed

Directions:

1. Combine pineapple, mango, coconut flakes, hemp seeds, and coconut milk in a blender
2. Blend until smooth
3. Add lime juice and ice cubes, blend until frosty

Tips:

- Add a pinch of turmeric for anti-inflammatory benefits
- Garnish with a few mint leaves for enhanced flavor and freshness

Nutritional Values: Calories: 210, Fat: 11g, Carbs: 28g, Protein: 3g, Sugar: 18g, Sodium: 30 mg, Potassium: 300 mg, Cholesterol: 0 mg

MINTY MELON REFRESH

Preparation Time: 8 min.

Cooking Time: none

Mode of Cooking: Blending

Servings: 2

Ingredients:

- 2 cups watermelon cubes
- 1/2 cucumber, sliced
- 12 fresh mint leaves
- 1 Tbsp lemon juice
- 1 Tbsp honey (optional, for non-Whole30)
- Ice cubes as needed

Directions:

1. Place watermelon, cucumber, mint leaves, and lemon juice in a blender

2. Blend until smooth
3. Add ice and blend to desired frostiness

Tips:

• Skip the honey for a Whole30 compliant version

• Serve immediately for best flavor and nutrient retention

Nutritional Values: Calories: 90, Fat: 0.5g, Carbs: 22g, Protein: 1g, Sugar: 18g (exclude if not adding honey), Sodium: 10 mg, Potassium: 270 mg, Cholesterol: 0 mg

GREEN DETOX POWER SMOOTHIE

Preparation Time: 10 min
Cooking Time: none
Mode of Cooking: Blending
Servings: 2
Ingredients:

• 1 cup fresh spinach
• 1 small cucumber, peeled and chopped
• 1 large ripe banana
• 1/2 avocado
• 1 Tbsp chia seeds
• 1 cup unsweetened almond milk
• 1 Tbsp fresh lemon juice
• handful of fresh parsley

Directions:

1. Combine all ingredients in a blender and blend on high until smooth
2. Pour into glasses and serve immediately

Tips:

• Add a piece of fresh ginger for an extra kick of flavor and digestive benefits

• If too thick, adjust consistency with a little more almond milk

Nutritional Values: Calories: 210, Fat: 11g, Carbs: 27g, Protein: 5g, Sugar: 11g, Sodium: 30 mg, Potassium: 487 mg, Cholesterol: 0 mg

• 3.2 WHOLESOME BOWLS

SAVORY SWEET POTATO & KALE BREAKFAST BOWL

Preparation Time: 10 min
Cooking Time: 20 min
Mode of Cooking: Stovetop
Servings: 2
Ingredients:

• 1 large sweet potato, peeled and diced
• 2 cups kale, chopped
• 4 eggs
• 1 avocado, sliced
• 2 Tbsp olive oil
• Sea salt and black pepper to taste
• 1 tsp smoked paprika
• ½ tsp garlic powder

Directions:

1. Heat olive oil in a skillet over medium heat
2. Add diced sweet potatoes and sauté until tender and golden, about 15 min
3. Stir in kale, smoked paprika, and garlic powder, cooking until kale is wilted, about 5 min
4. In another skillet, fry eggs to desired doneness
5. Assemble bowls by dividing sweet potato and kale mixture, topping each with two eggs and avocado slices

Tips:

• Add a pinch of red pepper flakes for a spicy kick

• Top with fresh herbs like cilantro or parsley for added freshness

Nutritional Values: Calories: 350, Fat: 22g, Carbs: 27g, Protein: 15g, Sugar: 3g, Sodium: 320 mg, Potassium: 847 mg, Cholesterol: 370 mg

COCONUT CAULIFLOWER RICE WITH PECANS AND BERRIES

Preparation Time: 15 min
Cooking Time: 10 min

Mode of Cooking: Stovetop

Servings: 2

Ingredients:

- 1 head of cauliflower, diced
- 1 cup coconut milk
- ½ cup pecans, chopped
- 1 cup mixed berries (blueberries, raspberries)
- 1 tsp cinnamon
- 2 Tbsp coconut oil
- Sprinkle of sea salt

Directions:

1. Heat coconut oil in a skillet over medium heat
2. Add diced cauliflower and a sprinkle of sea salt, cook until slightly tender, about 8 min
3. Stir in coconut milk and cinnamon, cook until absorbed, about 2 min
4. Remove from heat, mix in pecans and berries gently
5. Serve warm

Tips:

- Drizzle with a little honey if a touch of sweetness is desired
- Serve this bowl as a chilled dish for a refreshing breakfast option

Nutritional Values: Calories: 308, Fat: 24g, Carbs: 19g, Protein: 5g, Sugar: 8g, Sodium: 166 mg, Potassium: 730 mg, Cholesterol: 0 mg

SPICED CHICKEN & QUINOA BOWL

Preparation Time: 15 min.

Cooking Time: 25 min.

Mode of Cooking: Boiling/Sautéing

Servings: 3

Ingredients:

- 1 cup quinoa, rinsed
- 2 cups water
- 1 lb. chicken breast, cut into bite-sized pieces
- 1 tsp olive oil
- 1 red bell pepper, diced
- 1 zucchini, diced
- ½ tsp cumin
- ½ tsp coriander
- ½ tsp smoked paprika
- Salt and pepper to taste
- 2 Tbsp fresh cilantro, chopped
- 1 avocado, sliced
- 1 lime, cut into wedges

Directions:

1. Cook quinoa in water according to package instructions
2. heat olive oil in a pan over medium heat
3. sauté chicken pieces with salt, pepper, cumin, coriander, and paprika until golden and cooked through
4. add diced red bell pepper and zucchini to the pan in the last 5 min. of cooking
5. divide the quinoa among bowls
6. top with chicken, vegetables, fresh cilantro, and avocado slices
7. serve with lime wedges on the side

Tips:

- Use a rice cooker for quinoa for consistent results
- Adjust spice levels according to taste
- Add a drizzle of lime right before eating for extra zest

Nutritional Values: Calories: 495, Fat: 15g, Carbs: 52g, Protein: 36g, Sugar: 3g, Sodium: 85 mg, Potassium: 1250 mg, Cholesterol: 73 mg

HERBED TURKEY AND SPINACH BREAKFAST HASH

Preparation Time: 15 min

Cooking Time: 20 min

Mode of Cooking: Stovetop

Servings: 2

Ingredients:

- ½ lb ground turkey
- 2 cups spinach, chopped
- 1 large onion, chopped
- 2 cloves garlic, minced

- 2 Tbsp olive oil
- 1 tsp dried rosemary
- 1 tsp dried thyme
- Sea salt and black pepper to taste

Directions:

1. Heat olive oil in a large skillet over medium heat
2. Add chopped onion and minced garlic, sauté until onion is translucent
3. Add ground turkey, rosemary, thyme, salt, and pepper, cook until turkey is browned
4. Stir in spinach until wilted
5. Serve hot

Tips:

- Consider adding a poached egg on top for extra protein
- Mix in diced bell peppers for additional flavor and color

Nutritional Values: Calories: 295, Fat: 17g, Carbs: 7g, Protein: 28g, Sugar: 2g, Sodium: 75 mg, Potassium: 560 mg, Cholesterol: 80 mg

ALMOND BUTTER BANANA PROTEIN BOWL

Preparation Time: 5 min
Cooking Time: none
Mode of Cooking: No Cooking
Servings: 1
Ingredients:

- 1 banana, sliced
- ¼ cup almond butter
- ¼ cup walnuts, chopped
- 1 Tbsp chia seeds
- 1 tsp cinnamon
- ½ cup almond milk
- 1 scoop vanilla protein powder (Whole30 compliant)

Directions:

1. In a bowl, mix almond milk with protein powder until smooth
2. Add sliced bananas, almond butter, walnuts, and chia seeds

3. Sprinkle cinnamon on top
4. Stir gently to combine all ingredients

Tips:

- Experiment with different nut butters like cashew or peanut butter
- Add a dash of nutmeg for an extra flavor twist
- If you prefer a thinner consistency, add more almond milk

Nutritional Values: Calories: 410, Fat: 24g, Carbs: 34g, Protein: 18g, Sugar: 12g, Sodium: 110 mg, Potassium: 450 mg, Cholesterol: 10 mg

• 3.3 QUICK AND HEALTHY

CHIA AND COCONUT BREAKFAST PUDDING

Preparation Time: 15 min
Cooking Time: none
Mode of Cooking: No Cooking
Servings: 2
Ingredients:

- 1 C. coconut milk
- 1/4 C. chia seeds
- 1 tsp vanilla extract
- 1 Tbsp coconut flakes, unsweetened
- 1/2 C. mixed berries
- 1 Tbsp slivered almonds

Directions:

1. Combine coconut milk, chia seeds, and vanilla extract in a bowl and mix thoroughly
2. Cover and refrigerate overnight to set
3. In the morning, stir the set pudding, top with mixed berries, coconut flakes, and slivered almonds

Tips:

- Serve chilled for a refreshing start to the day
- Customize with different berries according to season
- Add a pinch of cinnamon for an extra flavor boost

Nutritional Values: Calories: 295, Fat: 21g, Carbs: 20g, Protein: 5g, Sugar: 5g, Sodium: 30 mg, Potassium: 150 mg, Cholesterol: 0 mg

SAVORY SPINACH AND MUSHROOM BREAKFAST CUPS

Preparation Time: 20 min
Cooking Time: 25 min
Mode of Cooking: Baking
Servings: 6
Ingredients:

- 6 eggs
- 1/2 C. fresh spinach, chopped
- 1/2 C. mushrooms, diced
- 1/4 C. onions, finely chopped
- 1 Tbsp olive oil
- Salt and pepper to taste

Directions:

1. Preheat oven to 350°F (175°C)
2. Sauté mushrooms and onions in olive oil until tender and golden
3. In a bowl, whisk eggs, salt, and pepper
4. Combine cooked vegetables and spinach with the egg mixture
5. Grease a muffin tin and evenly distribute the mixture into 6 cups
6. Bake for 25 min or until the egg cups are firm

Tips:

- Pairs well with a fresh arugula salad
- Store in the refrigerator for up to 3 days for a quick grab-and-go option

Nutritional Values: Calories: 120, Fat: 8g, Carbs: 3g, Protein: 9g, Sugar: 1g, Sodium: 125 mg, Potassium: 220 mg, Cholesterol: 185 mg

ALMOND FLOUR PANCAKES WITH FRESH BERRIES

Preparation Time: 10 min
Cooking Time: 15 min
Mode of Cooking: Pan Frying
Servings: 4

Ingredients:

- 1 C. almond flour
- 2 eggs
- 1/4 C. water
- 1 tsp vanilla extract
- 1 Tbsp coconut oil
- 1 C. fresh berries
- 1 Tbsp honey (optional, omit for Whole30 compliance)

Directions:

1. Mix almond flour, eggs, water, and vanilla extract until smooth
2. Heat coconut oil in a skillet over medium heat
3. Pour batter to form small pancakes, cook until bubbles appear, then flip and cook until golden brown
4. Serve with fresh berries and a drizzle of honey if desired

Tips:

- Make a large batch and freeze for easy weekday breakfasts
- Use a variety of berries for different flavors and nutrients

Nutritional Values: Calories: 250, Fat: 18g, Carbs: 12g, Protein: 9g, Sugar: 6g (0g if honey is omitted), Sodium: 45 mg, Potassium: 100 mg, Cholesterol: 90 mg

AVOCADO AND EGG TOAST WITH RADISH

Preparation Time: 5 min
Cooking Time: 5 min
Mode of Cooking: Pan Frying
Servings: 2
Ingredients:

- 2 slices sweet potato (thick cut)
- 1 avocado
- 2 eggs
- 4 radishes, thinly sliced
- Salt and pepper to taste
- 1 Tbsp ghee

Directions:

1. Toast sweet potato slices in a toaster or oven until crisp
2. Fry eggs in ghee to desired consistency
3. Mash avocado and spread on toasted sweet potato slices
4. Top with fried eggs and radish slices
5. Season with salt and pepper

Tips:

● This dish is high in healthy fats and a perfect quick meal

● Enhance flavor by sprinkling with crushed red pepper flakes or smoked paprika

Nutritional Values: Calories: 320, Fat: 24g, Carbs: 18g, Protein: 10g, Sugar: 4g, Sodium: 65 mg, Potassium: 700 mg, Cholesterol: 185 mg

SPICED CHIA AND COCONUT BREAKFAST PUDDING

Preparation Time: 10 min

Cooking Time: none

Mode of Cooking: No Cooking

Servings: 2

Ingredients:

● 1 C. coconut milk
● 3 Tbsp chia seeds
● 1 tsp cinnamon
● ½ tsp nutmeg
● 1 Tbsp almond butter
● 2 tsp vanilla extract
● Optional toppings: sliced almonds, unsweetened coconut flakes, fresh berries

Directions:

1. Combine coconut milk, chia seeds, cinnamon, nutmeg, almond butter, and vanilla extract in a bowl
2. Stir thoroughly until well mixed
3. Let the mixture sit for 10 min to allow chia seeds to swell and create a pudding-like consistency
4. Serve with optional toppings as desired

Tips:

● Overnight Option: Prepare the night before and let it sit in the refrigerator for an easy grab-and-go breakfast

● Personalize with different toppings like nuts, seeds, and seasonal fruits to vary the flavours and textures

Nutritional Values: Calories: 295, Fat: 25g, Carbs: 15g, Protein: 5g, Sugar: 3g, Sodium: 30 mg, Potassium: 200 mg, Cholesterol: 0 mg

CHAPTER 4: LUNCH DELIGHTS

Imagine this: It's the middle of your bustling day, the clock strikes noon, and your energy dips just as deadlines loom and meetings stack up. The temptation to grab a quick bag of chips or order a greasy burger for lunch tugs at you. But what if, instead, you could invigorate your afternoon with a plate full of vibrant, wholesome foods that not only satisfy your hunger but also boost your energy levels and keep you on track with your health goals?

Welcome to the heartwarming world of Lunch Delights, where each recipe is a celebration of nutritious ingredients that come together to keep you nourished and motivated through your workday. Think of lunches that combine simplicity with nutrition, peppered with flavors that make each noon-time meal a delightful experience. Picture yourself unwrapping a roasted vegetable and quinoa wrap, the vegetables brightly caramelized and the grains giving you that perfect punch of protein.

Or perhaps on a chillier day, a bowl of fragrant, homemade soup awaits you; its steam carrying the aroma of fresh herbs and robust spices that promise to comfort as much as they heal. These meals aren't just about filling up but rejuvenating your body and mind amidst daily challenges.

Within this chapter, we bypass the mundane and uplift the simple act of eating lunch to a nourishing ritual. This isn't about overhauling your entire diet but introducing accessible, delicious changes that make a sizable impact. As you explore these pages filled with salads bursting with colors, wraps packed with layers of texture, and soups that tell a story of cultural heritage and culinary love, remember each recipe is crafted keeping in mind your busy schedule and your family's diverse palates.

Embark on this flavorful journey where each lunch is a step toward sustained health and well-being, proving that even in your busiest moments, feeding your body with whole, satiating foods is not only possible but also a delightful indulgence.

• 4.1 FRESH AND FILLING

TAHINI KALE SALAD WITH ROASTED CHICKPEAS

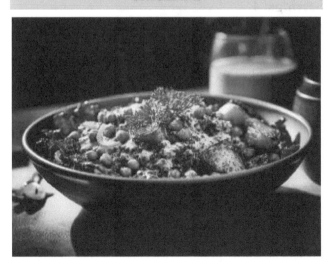

Preparation Time: 20 min.
Cooking Time: 25 min.

Mode of Cooking: Roasting, Tossing
Servings: 4
Ingredients:

- 1 bunch kale, stems removed and leaves torn
- 1 can chickpeas, drained and rinsed
- 2 Tbsp olive oil
- 1 tsp smoked paprika
- Salt and black pepper to taste
- 1 small red onion, thinly sliced
- 1/4 cup tahini
- 2 Tbsp lemon juice
- 1 garlic clove, minced
- 5 radishes, thinly sliced
- 1/4 cup pumpkin seeds

Directions:

1. Preheat oven to 425°F (220°C)
2. In a bowl, toss chickpeas with 1 Tbsp olive oil, smoked paprika, salt, and black pepper
3. Spread on a baking sheet and roast for 20 min. until crispy
4. Massage kale with remaining olive oil and a pinch of salt until leaves are tender
5. In a small bowl, whisk together tahini, lemon juice, garlic, and 3 Tbsp water to make a dressing
6. Combine kale, roasted chickpeas, red onion, radishes, and pumpkin seeds in a serving bowl
7. Drizzle with tahini dressing and toss to combine

Tips:

● Addition of avocado provides extra creaminess and healthy fats

● Massage the kale leaves thoroughly to make them softer and easier to digest

● Serve immediately to enjoy the crunch of chickpeas

Nutritional Values: Calories: 297, Fat: 17g, Carbs: 29g, Protein: 9g, Sugar: 4g, Sodium: 210 mg, Potassium: 448 mg, Cholesterol: 0 mg

QUINOA BEET SALAD WITH ORANGE VINAIGRETTE

Preparation Time: 15 min.

Cooking Time: none

Mode of Cooking: Mixing

Servings: 4

Ingredients:

● 1 cup quinoa, cooked

● 2 medium beets, roasted and diced

● 1/4 cup walnuts, chopped

● 1/4 cup crumbled feta cheese (omit for Whole30)

● 1 orange, juiced

● 2 Tbsp olive oil

● 1 Tbsp balsamic vinegar

● Salt and black pepper to taste

● 1/4 cup chopped parsley

Directions:

1. In a large bowl, combine cooked quinoa, beets, walnuts, and feta cheese
2. In a separate small bowl, whisk together orange juice, olive oil, balsamic vinegar, salt, and pepper to create the vinaigrette
3. Pour the vinaigrette over the quinoa mixture and toss until well combined
4. Sprinkle with chopped parsley just before serving

Tips:

● Toast walnuts briefly in a dry pan for extra flavor and crunch

● Orange zest can be added to the vinaigrette for a more vibrant flavor

● This salad can be served either warm or chilled, making it versatile for all seasons

Nutritional Values: Calories: 315, Fat: 15g, Carbs: 38g, Protein: 8g, Sugar: 7g, Sodium: 180 mg, Potassium: 520 mg, Cholesterol: 10 mg

SPICY SWEET POTATO & BLACK BEAN BOWL

Preparation Time: 15 min.

Cooking Time: 25 min.

Mode of Cooking: Boiling, Sauteing

Servings: 4

Ingredients:

● 2 large sweet potatoes, peeled and cubed

● 1 can black beans, rinsed and drained

● 1 Tbsp coconut oil

● 1 tsp cumin

● 1/2 tsp chili powder

● Salt and black pepper

● 2 cloves garlic

● pepper to taste

● 1 small avocado, diced

● 1 lime, juiced

● 1/4 cup fresh cilantro, chopped

Directions:

1. Boil sweet potatoes in salted water until tender, about 15 min.
2. Drain and set aside
3. Heat coconut oil in a pan over medium heat
4. Add cumin, chili powder, and drained sweet potatoes and sauté for 5 min. until lightly crispy
5. Add black beans and cook until heated thoroughly
6. Remove from heat and add avocado
7. add salt, lime juice, and cilantro
8. Mix well and serve immediately

Tips:

● Serve with a dollop of cashew cream for added richness

● Including jalapeno or your favorite hot sauce can intensify the spiciness according to your taste

● Lime zest can be included to enhance citrus notes

Nutritional Values: Calories: 256, Fat: 7g, Carbs: 43g, Protein: 7g, Sugar: 6g, Sodium: 239 mg, Potassium: 676 mg, Cholesterol: 0 mg

MEDITERRANEAN CAULIFLOWER TABBOULEH

Preparation Time: 20 min.

Cooking Time: 10 min.

Mode of Cooking: Boiling, Chopping

Servings: 4

Ingredients:

● 1 head cauliflower, riced
● 1 cup cherry tomatoes, halved
● 1 cucumber, diced
● 1/2 cup parsley, finely chopped
● 1/4 cup mint, finely chopped
● 1 lemon, juiced
● 2 Tbsp olive oil
● Salt and black pepper
● Chopped dill, for garnish
● 1 clove garlic, minced

Directions:

1. Boil riced cauliflower in salted water for 5 min. just until tender
2. Drain and let cool
3. In a large bowl, combine cooled cauliflower, cherry tomatoes, cucumber, parsley, mint, lemon juice, olive oil, garlic, and salt and pepper
4. Toss to combine
5. Garnish with chopped dill before serving

Tips:

● Add crumbled feta cheese for extra flavor (omit for Whole30)

● A sprinkle of sumac can add a tangy zest to the dish

● Chill before serving to allow flavors to meld together beautifully

Nutritional Values: Calories: 123, Fat: 7g, Carbs: 14g, Protein: 4g, Sugar: 5g, Sodium: 67 mg, Potassium: 467 mg, Cholesterol: 0 mg

RAINBOW VEGETABLE NICOISE SALAD

Preparation Time: 20 min.

Cooking Time: none

Mode of Cooking: No Cooking

Servings: 4

Ingredients:

● 2 heads of Boston lettuce, leaves separated and washed
● 4 small radishes, thinly sliced
● 1 small red onion, thinly sliced
● 2 large ripe tomatoes, cut into wedges
● 1 cucumber, sliced into half-moons
● 12 small new potatoes, boiled and halved
● 2 Tbsp capers, rinsed
● 12 oz. green beans, blanched
● 4 hard-boiled eggs, peeled and quartered
● 12 oz. fresh grilled tuna, flaked
● 1 lemon, juiced
● 6 Tbsp extra virgin olive oil
● 2 tsp Dijon mustard

- Salt and pepper to taste

Directions:

1. Arrange lettuce leaves at the bottom of a large platter
2. scatter radishes, red onion, tomatoes, and cucumber over lettuce
3. arrange potatoes, green beans, and eggs in sections around the vegetables
4. scatter tuna and capers over the top
5. whisk together lemon juice, olive oil, mustard, salt, and pepper to create the dressing
6. pour dressing evenly over the salad just before serving

Tips:

- Prepare ingredients ahead to save time
- Customize with different seasonal vegetables for variety
- Use high-quality olive oil for the best flavor

Nutritional Values: Calories: 380, Fat: 22g, Carbs: 28g, Protein: 24g, Sugar: 5g, Sodium: 220 mg, Potassium: 980 mg, Cholesterol: 190 mg

4.2 WRAPS AND SANDWICHES

AVOCADO & SMOKED SALMON LETTUCE WRAPS

Preparation Time: 15 min

Cooking Time: none

Mode of Cooking: No Cooking

Servings: 2

Ingredients:

- 1 large avocado, peeled and sliced
- 4 oz. smoked salmon, thinly sliced
- 1 small red onion, thinly sliced
- 1 Tbsp capers
- 1 Tbsp fresh dill, chopped
- 6 large lettuce leaves, preferably Bibb or Butter lettuce
- 1 tsp fresh lemon juice
- Sea salt and black pepper to taste

Directions:

1. Place lettuce leaves on a flat surface
2. Lay slices of smoked salmon on each lettuce leaf
3. In a bowl, mix sliced avocado with lemon juice, sea salt, and black pepper
4. Place seasoned avocado slices on top of the salmon
5. Garnish each wrap with red onion slices, capers, and fresh dill
6. Carefully fold the lettuce leaves to form wraps

Tips:

- Opt for high-quality smoked salmon for better flavor and texture
- Squeeze lemon juice over the avocado to prevent browning
- These wraps can be customized with other fresh herbs like cilantro or parsley

Nutritional Values: Calories: 300, Fat: 22g, Carbs: 9g, Protein: 15g, Sugar: 2g, Sodium: 600 mg, Potassium: 650 mg, Cholesterol: 20 mg

SPICY TURKEY & CUCUMBER NORI ROLLS

Preparation Time: 20 min

Cooking Time: none

Mode of Cooking: No Cooking

Servings: 4

Ingredients:

- 8 oz. turkey breast, thinly sliced
- 1 medium cucumber, julienned
- 1 carrot, julienne
- 2 Tbsp Sriracha sauce
- 4 nori seaweed sheets
- 1 Tbsp sesame seeds
- 1 avocado, sliced
- 1 tsp soy sauce (ensure Whole30 compliance)
- 1 tsp wasabi paste (optional)

Directions:

1. Lay out nori sheets on a bamboo sushi mat

2. Spread Sriracha sauce lightly across each nori sheet
3. Arrange turkey slices along the edge of each nori sheet
4. Add julienned cucumber and carrot strips over the turkey
5. Add avocado slices next to the vegetables
6. Roll the nori tightly using the bamboo mat, starting from the edge with the fillers towards the empty side
7. Slice each roll into six pieces
8. Drizzle with a mix of soy sauce and wasabi paste for added flavor if desired

Tips:

• Use a sharp knife to cut the rolls to prevent tearing the nori

• Wet the knife slightly between cuts for cleaner slices

• Serve immediately or keep refrigerated until ready to eat

Nutritional Values: Calories: 180, Fat: 6g, Carbs: 12g, Protein: 20g, Sugar: 3g, Sodium: 420 mg, Potassium: 300 mg, Cholesterol: 30 mg

ALMOND BUTTER & BANANA CHIA SEED SANDWICH

Preparation Time: 10 min
Cooking Time: none
Mode of Cooking: No Cooking
Servings: 2
Ingredients:

• 2 Tbsp almond butter
• 1 medium banana, sliced
• 1 Tbsp chia seeds
• 4 slices of Whole30-compliant bread
• 1 Tbsp raw honey (omit for Whole30 version)
• Cinnamon to taste

Directions:

1. Spread almond butter evenly on two slices of bread

2. Place sliced banana on top of the almond butter
3. Sprinkle chia seeds and cinnamon over the banana slices
4. Drizzle honey if not following Whole30
5. Top with the remaining slices of bread to make two sandwiches

Tips:

• Try toasting the bread slightly for a crunchier texture

• Add a sprinkle of nutmeg for an extra flavor boost if desired

• Ensure all ingredients are compliant with Whole30 guidelines if following that dietary plan

Nutritional Values: Calories: 350, Fat: 18g, Carbs: 40g, Protein: 8g, Sugar: 12g (omit if following Whole30), Sodium: 200 mg, Potassium: 300 mg, Cholesterol: 0 mg

CHICKEN CAESAR HEMP SEED WRAP

Preparation Time: 25 min
Cooking Time: none
Mode of Cooking: No Cooking
Servings: 2
Ingredients:

• 2 cups cooked chicken breast, shredded
• 2 large collard greens, stems trimmed
• 1/4 cup Caesar dressing (Whole30-compliant)
• 1/4 cup hemp seeds
• 1/4 cup shredded Parmesan cheese (omit for Whole30 version)
• Freshly ground black pepper to taste

Directions:

1. Blanch collard greens for 30 seconds in boiling water, then cool in ice water
2. Pat dry the greens
3. Lay out collard greens on a clean surface
4. Spread Caesar dressing over the greens
5. Top with shredded chicken, hemp seeds, and Parmesan cheese if not following Whole30
6. Season with black pepper

7. Roll up tightly, tucking in the edges as you go

Tips:

● Blanching the collard greens makes them more pliable and easier to wrap

● If avoiding dairy, replace Parmesan with nutritional yeast for a cheesy flavor

● Serve with additional Caesar dressing on the side for dipping

Nutritional Values: Calories: 410, Fat: 22g, Carbs: 4g, Protein: 44g, Sugar: 1g, Sodium: 590 mg, Potassium: 400 mg, Cholesterol: 100 mg

TAHINI CHICKPEA WRAP WITH AVOCADO AND SPINACH

Preparation Time: 15 min

Cooking Time: none

Mode of Cooking: No Cooking

Servings: 2

Ingredients:

● 2 large collard greens leaves, stems trimmed

● 1 cup cooked chickpeas

● 1 medium avocado, sliced

● 1 small carrot, shredded

● 1/2 cup baby spinach

● 1/4 cup red onion, thinly sliced

● 2 Tbsp tahini

● 1 Tbsp lemon juice

● 1 tsp garlic powder

● Salt and pepper to taste

Directions:

1. Wash and pat dry collard greens leaves
2. In a small bowl, mix tahini, lemon juice, garlic powder, salt, and pepper until smooth
3. Spread tahini mixture over each collard leaf
4. Top with chickpeas, avocado slices, shredded carrot, baby spinach, and red onion
5. Roll up tightly, starting at one end, tucking in sides as you roll

Tips:

● Use a toothpick to secure wraps if needed

● For extra flavor, include a sprinkle of crushed red pepper flakes or cumin in the tahini sauce

● Can substitute collard greens with any large leafy green like kale or chard

Nutritional Values: Calories: 265, Fat: 15g, Carbs: 28g, Protein: 9g, Sugar: 3g, Sodium: 45 mg, Potassium: 846 mg, Cholesterol: 0 mg

• 4.3 SOUPS AND STEWS

HEARTY BEEF AND VEGETABLE STEW

Preparation Time: 20 min.

Cooking Time: 1 hr. 30 min.

Mode of Cooking: Stovetop

Servings: 6

Ingredients:

● 2 lb. lean beef chuck, cut into cubes

● 3 Tbsp olive oil

● 2 large carrots, sliced

● 2 stalks celery, chopped

● 1 large onion, diced

● 4 cloves garlic, minced

● 2 Tbsp tomato paste

● 1 qt. beef broth

● 1 cup water

● 1 Tbsp dried thyme

● 1 bay leaf

● 2 cups diced potatoes

● Salt and pepper to taste

Directions:

1. Heat the olive oil in a large pot over medium heat, add beef cubes and brown on all sides
2. Remove beef and set aside
3. In the same pot, add onions, carrots, and celery, cook until softened
4. Add garlic and cook for another minute
5. Return beef to the pot along with tomato paste, stir for 2 min.
6. Pour in beef broth and water, add thyme and bay leaf

7. Bring to a boil, then reduce to a simmer, cover, and cook for 1 hr.
8. Add potatoes and cook uncovered for an additional 30 min. or until potatoes are tender

Tips:
- Stir occasionally to prevent sticking
- Skim off any excess fat during simmering process
- Can be served with a side of steamed vegetables for added nutrition

Nutritional Values: Calories: 350, Fat: 15g, Carbs: 22g, Protein: 28g, Sugar: 5g, Sodium: 470 mg, Potassium: 940 mg, Cholesterol: 90 mg

SPICY TOMATO AND SHRIMP SOUP

Preparation Time: 15 min.
Cooking Time: 25 min.
Mode of Cooking: Stovetop
Servings: 4
Ingredients:
- 1 Tbsp coconut oil
- 1 onion, chopped
- 2 cloves garlic, minced
- 1 tsp smoked paprika
- 1/2 tsp cayenne pepper
- 1 Tbsp tomato paste
- 1 qt. vegetable broth
- 1 lb. fresh shrimp, peeled and deveined
- 1 cup diced tomatoes
- 2 Tbsp chopped fresh parsley
- Salt and pepper to taste

Directions:

1. Heat the coconut oil in a large pot over medium heat
2. Add onion and garlic, sauté until soft
3. Stir in smoked paprika, cayenne pepper, and tomato paste, cook for 1 min.
4. Pour in vegetable broth, bring to a boil
5. Add shrimp and tomatoes, reduce heat and simmer for 15 min. or until shrimp are cooked through

6. Season with salt and pepper, garnish with fresh parsley before serving

Tips:
- Serve hot and adjust seasoning as necessary
- Great with a slice of toasted gluten-free bread
- Shrimp can be substituted with chicken for a different flavor profile

Nutritional Values: Calories: 180, Fat: 6g, Carbs: 12g, Protein: 20g, Sugar: 5g, Sodium: 800 mg, Potassium: 300 mg, Cholesterol: 115 mg

CURRIED COCONUT CHICKEN SOUP

Preparation Time: 10 min.
Cooking Time: 40 min.
Mode of Cooking: Stovetop
Servings: 4
Ingredients:
- 1 Tbsp olive oil
- 1 lb. chicken breast, cut into strips
- 1 onion, diced
- 2 Tbsp grated ginger
- 4 cloves garlic, minced
- 2 Tbsp curry powder
- 1 can (14 oz.) coconut milk
- 1 qt. chicken broth
- 1 red bell pepper, sliced
- 1 cup chopped spinach
- Salt to taste

Directions:

1. Heat olive oil in a large pot over medium heat
2. Add chicken and cook until browned on all sides
3. Remove chicken and set aside
4. In the same pot, add onion, ginger, and garlic, sauté for 5 min.
5. Stir in curry powder and cook for 1 min.
6. Return chicken to the pot, add coconut milk and chicken broth
7. Bring to a boil, then simmer for 30 min.
8. Add red bell pepper and spinach, cook for an additional 10 min.

Tips:

- Add fresh lime juice for a zestier flavor
- Use full-fat coconut milk for richer taste and texture
- Serve with cauli-rice for a complete meal

Nutritional Values: Calories: 295, Fat: 15g, Carbs: 10g, Protein: 28g, Sugar: 3g, Sodium: 870 mg, Potassium: 540 mg, Cholesterol: 60 mg

RUSTIC MUSHROOM AND BARLEY SOUP

Preparation Time: 10 min.

Cooking Time: 1 hr.

Mode of Cooking: Stovetop

Servings: 6

Ingredients:

- 2 Tbsp ghee
- 1 lb. mixed mushrooms, sliced
- 1 onion, diced
- 2 carrots, diced
- 2 stalks celery, diced
- 4 cloves garlic, minced
- 1 cup pearl barley
- 6 cups vegetable broth
- 2 tsp dried thyme
- Salt and pepper to taste

Directions:

1. Heat ghee in a large pot over medium heat
2. Add mushrooms, onion, carrots, celery, and garlic, cook until vegetables are soft, about 10 min.
3. Stir in barley, cook for 1 min.
4. Add vegetable broth and thyme
5. Bring to a boil, then reduce to a simmer, cover, and cook for 50 min. or until barley is tender

Tips:

- Serve warm sprinkled with fresh parsley
- Ideal for batch cooking and freezes well
- Enhance flavor with a splash of low sodium soy sauce

Nutritional Values: Calories: 200, Fat: 7g, Carbs: 30g, Protein: 8g, Sugar: 5g, Sodium: 300 mg, Potassium: 400 mg, Cholesterol: 15 mg

SPICY TOMATO AND SHRIMP STEW

Preparation Time: 15 min.

Cooking Time: 30 min.

Mode of Cooking: Stovetop

Servings: 4

Ingredients:

- 2 Tbsp olive oil
- 1 lb. shrimp, peeled and deveined
- 1 large onion, finely chopped
- 3 garlic cloves, minced
- 1 tsp smoked paprika
- 1/2 tsp red pepper flakes
- 1 can (14 oz.) whole tomatoes, crushed by hand
- 1 cup fish broth
- 1 tsp sea salt
- 1/4 tsp freshly ground black pepper
- Fresh parsley, chopped, for garnish

Directions:

1. Heat olive oil in a large pot over medium heat
2. Add the onions and garlic, sauté until translucent, about 5 minutes
3. Add the smoked paprika and red pepper flakes, stir to combine
4. Add crushed tomatoes and fish broth, bring to a simmer
5. Add the shrimp and cook until they are pink and opaque, about 8-10 minutes
6. Season with salt and pepper
7. Garnish with fresh parsley

Tips:

- Serve with a side of steamed vegetables to enhance the nutrients in your meal
- Consider adding a spoonful of almond butter for a richer, nutty flavor in the stew

Nutritional Values: Calories: 210, Fat: 8g, Carbs: 12g, Protein: 20g, Sugar: 4g, Sodium: 720 mg, Potassium: 350 mg, Cholesterol: 115 mg

CHAPTER 5: DINNER RECIPES

As the sun dips below the horizon and the busy day winds down, there's nothing quite like gathering around the dinner table to share a meal that not only satisfies the stomach but also nourishes the soul. Dinner is more than just a meal; it's a moment to reconnect with loved ones, to share stories of the day, and to rejuvenate with dishes that are as nurturing as they are delightful.

In the realm of whole foods, dinner becomes an opportunity to explore a world of flavors without straying from the path of health. Imagine sitting down to a dish where every ingredient offers a bounty of nutrients, where the natural flavors of vegetables, grains, and proteins meld together in a symphony of taste and wellness. This isn't just food; it's a celebration of life's simple pleasures.

Here, in this chapter, we embark on a culinary adventure with dinner recipes that promise ease and excitement. Picture a One-Dish Wonder that requires minimal cleanup yet bursts with the savory aromas of herbs and spices. Envision preparing a Roasted and Baked masterpiece that transforms the humblest of vegetables into a centerpiece worthy of a feast. And when comfort calls, a heartwarming casserole or slow-cooked favorite provides the perfect answer to your craving for coziness.

Each recipe is crafted with the beginner in mind, ensuring that even those new to the kitchen can achieve success. The ingredients list remains uncomplicated, the steps are straightforward, and the results? Absolutely satisfying. But beyond the simplicity, these meals are designed to be flexible, allowing you to experiment with substitutions and add your twists depending on what's fresh and available.

By the end of this chapter, my hope is that you'll not only have a collection of recipes to turn to but also the confidence to view dinner as a time for creativity and healthful indulgence. Whether a quiet meal for one or a bustling feast for many, these dinner ideas are here to ensure that every evening meal enriches your body, delights your palate, and brings joy to your table.

• 5.1 ONE-DISH WONDERS

TURMERIC COCONUT BRAISED CHICKEN

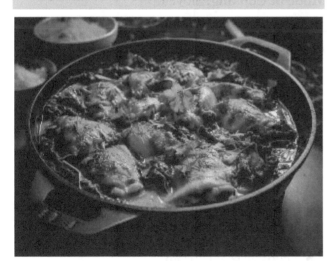

Preparation Time: 15 min
Cooking Time: 1 hr
Mode of Cooking: Stovetop

Servings: 4
Ingredients:
- 4 bone-in, skin-on chicken thighs
- 1 large onion, thinly sliced
- 4 cloves garlic, minced
- 1 Tbsp freshly grated turmeric
- 1 Tbsp ground coriander
- 1 tsp cumin seeds
- 400 ml coconut milk
- 1 bunch kale, stems removed and leaves chopped
- Salt and pepper to taste
- 2 Tbsp coconut oil

Directions:

1. Heat coconut oil in a large pot over medium heat
2. Add onions and garlic, sauté until translucent
3. Stir in turmeric, coriander, and cumin seeds, cook for 1 min
4. Place chicken thighs skin-side down, cook until browned on each side, approximately 5 min per side
5. Pour in coconut milk and bring to a boil
6. Reduce heat to low, cover, and simmer for 45 min
7. Add chopped kale in the last 10 min of cooking
8. Season with salt and pepper

Tips:

- Use a heavy lid to keep the steam in for more tenderness
- Serve hot directly from the pot to keep flavors intact
- Pair with cauliflower rice for a complete Whole30 dish

Nutritional Values: Calories: 450, Fat: 30g, Carbs: 12g, Protein: 30g, Sugar: 2g, Sodium: 150 mg, Potassium: 500 mg, Cholesterol: 120 mg

SPICY SHRIMP AND ANDOUILLE SAUSAGE SKILLET

Preparation Time: 10 min
Cooking Time: 20 min
Mode of Cooking: Stovetop
Servings: 4
Ingredients:

- 300g andouille sausage, sliced
- 500g shrimp, peeled and deveined
- 1 bell pepper, diced
- 1 onion, diced
- 2 cloves garlic, minced
- 1 tsp smoked paprika
- 1/2 tsp chili flakes
- 400g diced tomatoes, no salt added

- 2 Tbsp olive oil
- Fresh parsley for garnish

Directions:

1. Heat olive oil in a large skillet over medium heat
2. Add sausage and cook until browned
3. Add bell pepper, onion, and garlic, sauté until soft
4. Stir in paprika and chili flakes
5. Add shrimp and cook until pink, about 3-5 min
6. Pour in diced tomatoes and simmer for 10 min
7. Garnish with fresh parsley

Tips:

- Cook shrimp separately if preferred less spicy
- Can substitute chicken for shrimp if desired
- Add a splash of chicken broth for more sauce if dry

Nutritional Values: Calories: 320, Fat: 18g, Carbs: 10g, Protein: 25g, Sugar: 5g, Sodium: 800 mg, Potassium: 300 mg, Cholesterol: 180 mg

MEDITERRANEAN LAMB STEW

Preparation Time: 20 min
Cooking Time: 2 hr
Mode of Cooking: Stovetop
Servings: 6
Ingredients:

- 1.5 lb lamb shoulder, cut into chunks
- 1 large onion, chopped
- 4 cloves garlic, minced
- 1 fennel bulb, chopped
- 3 carrots, peeled and sliced
- 1 tsp dried rosemary
- 1 tsp dried thyme
- 1 cup diced tomatoes
- 4 cups vegetable broth
- 2 Tbsp olive oil
- Salt and pepper to taste

Directions:

1. Heat olive oil in a heavy-bottomed pot over medium-high heat
2. Brown lamb chunks on all sides and set aside ♪ Sauté onions, garlic, fennel, and carrots until soft ♫ Return lamb to the pot, add rosemary, thyme, tomatoes, and broth ♪ Bring to a boil, then reduce heat and simmer covered for 1.5 to 2 hrs until lamb is tender ♫ Season with salt and pepper

Tips:

- Use lamb leg if shoulder not available
- Stir occasionally to prevent sticking
- Serve with fresh herbs for enhanced flavor

Nutritional Values: Calories: 350, Fat: 22g, Carbs: 15g, Protein: 25g, Sugar: 6g, Sodium: 600 mg, Potassium: 850 mg, Cholesterol: 80 mg

AUTUMN VEGETABLE BAKE

Preparation Time: 10 min

Cooking Time: 45 min

Mode of Cooking: Oven

Servings: 4

Ingredients:

- 3 sweet potatoes, peeled and cubed
- 2 parsnips, peeled and sliced
- 1 butternut squash, peeled and cubed
- 1 large onion, chopped
- 3 Tbsp olive oil
- 1 tsp cinnamon
- 1/2 tsp nutmeg
- Salt and pepper to taste
- Fresh thyme for garnish

Directions:

1. Preheat oven to 375°F (190°C)
2. In a large bowl, toss sweet potatoes, parsnips, butternut squash, and onion with olive oil, cinnamon, nutmeg, salt, and pepper
3. Spread evenly on a baking sheet
4. Bake for 45 min or until vegetables are tender and slightly caramelized

5. Garnish with fresh thyme

Tips:

- Mix root vegetables for different flavors
- Line baking sheet with parchment for easy cleanup
- Drizzle with balsamic glaze before serving for added zest

Nutritional Values: Calories: 210, Fat: 7g, Carbs: 35g, Protein: 2g, Sugar: 8g, Sodium: 75 mg, Potassium: 600 mg, Cholesterol: 0 mg

RUSTIC CHICKEN & ROOT VEGETABLE BAKE

Preparation Time: 15 min.

Cooking Time: 1 hr. 10 min.

Mode of Cooking: Baking

Servings: 4

Ingredients:

- 2 lb. bone-in, skin-on chicken thighs
- 1 lb. carrots, peeled and cut into chunks
- 1 lb. parsnips, peeled and cut into chunks
- 2 large onions, peeled and quartered
- 6 cloves garlic, peeled
- 3 Tbsp olive oil
- 2 tsp. smoked paprika
- 1 tsp. dried thyme
- Sea salt and freshly ground black pepper to taste

Directions:

1. Preheat oven to 375°F (190°C)
2. In a large bowl, toss the chicken and vegetables with olive oil, smoked paprika, thyme, salt, and pepper until well coated
3. Spread evenly on a large roasting pan or Dutch oven
4. Roast in the oven, stirring occasionally, until chicken is golden and vegetables are tender, about 70 minutes

Tips:

- Rotate the pan halfway through for even cooking

- Let rest for 5 minutes before serving to allow juices to redistribute

Nutritional Values: Calories: 620, Fat: 35g, Carbs: 34g, Protein: 45g, Sugar: 10g, Sodium: 300 mg, Potassium: 1050 mg, Cholesterol: 220 mg

---

• 5.2 ROASTED AND BAKED

HARISSA-RUBBED BAKED TROUT

Preparation Time: 15 min

Cooking Time: 20 min

Mode of Cooking: Baking

Servings: 4

Ingredients:

- 4 whole trout, cleaned and gutted
- 3 Tbsp olive oil
- 2 Tbsp harissa paste
- 2 tsp minced garlic
- 1 Tbsp lemon zest
- 1 lemon, thinly sliced
- Salt and freshly ground black pepper to taste
- Fresh parsley for garnishing

Directions:

1. Preheat oven to 375°F (190°C)
2. In a bowl, mix olive oil, harissa paste, minced garlic, lemon zest, salt, and black pepper
3. Rub this mixture both inside and outside the trout
4. Place lemon slices inside the cavity of each trout
5. Arrange trout on a lined baking sheet
6. Bake in the preheated oven until the fish flakes easily with a fork, about 20 min
7. Garnish with fresh parsley before serving

Tips:

- Use gloves when applying harissa to avoid skin irritation

- Serve with a side of roasted vegetables such as asparagus or carrots

Nutritional Values: Calories: 280, Fat: 15g, Carbs: 1g, Protein: 34g, Sugar: 0g, Sodium: 75mg, Potassium: 560mg, Cholesterol: 90mg

SPICED CAULIFLOWER AND CHICKPEA BAKE

Preparation Time: 10 min

Cooking Time: 40 min

Mode of Cooking: Baking

Servings: 6

Ingredients:

- 1 large head cauliflower, cut into florets
- 2 cans chickpeas, drained and rinsed
- 3 Tbsp olive oil
- 2 tsp smoked paprika
- 1 tsp ground cumin
- 1/2 tsp turmeric
- Salt and black pepper to taste
- 1/4 cup chopped fresh cilantro
- 1/4 cup sliced almonds

Directions:

1. Preheat oven to 400°F (200°C)
2. In a large bowl, combine olive oil, smoked paprika, ground cumin, turmeric, salt, and black pepper
3. Add cauliflower florets and chickpeas, toss to coat thoroughly
4. Spread the mixture on a baking sheet in a single layer
5. Bake for 40 min, stirring halfway through, until cauliflower is tender and slightly crispy
6. Sprinkle with chopped cilantro and sliced almonds before serving

Tips:

- For added crunch, roast the almonds before sprinkling them on top

- Consider adding a dollop of dairy-free yogurt to serve

Nutritional Values: Calories: 220, Fat: 10g, Carbs: 28g, Protein: 9g, Sugar: 5g, Sodium: 300mg, Potassium: 482mg, Cholesterol: 0mg

ROSEMARY LEMON BAKED CHICKEN THIGHS

Preparation Time: 10 min

Cooking Time: 45 min

Mode of Cooking: Baking

Servings: 4

Ingredients:

- 8 chicken thighs, bone-in and skin-on
- 4 Tbsp olive oil
- 4 cloves garlic, minced
- 1 Tbsp fresh rosemary, chopped
- 2 lemons, 1 juiced and 1 sliced
- Salt and black pepper to taste
- 1 tsp red pepper flakes

Directions:

1. Preheat oven to 425°F (220°C)
2. In a small bowl, mix olive oil, garlic, rosemary, lemon juice, salt, black pepper, and red pepper flakes
3. Place chicken thighs on a baking tray and rub them thoroughly with the marinade
4. Arrange lemon slices among the chicken thighs
5. Roast in the preheated oven until the chicken is golden and cooked through, about 45 min
6. Baste occasionally with pan juices during cooking

Tips:

- Brining the chicken for a few hours beforehand can enhance moisture and flavor
- Roast with additional fresh rosemary sprigs to intensify the aroma

Nutritional Values: Calories: 410, Fat: 31g, Carbs: 3g, Protein: 30g, Sugar: 1g, Sodium: 85mg, Potassium: 340mg, Cholesterol: 180mg

BALSAMIC ROASTED ROOT VEGETABLES

Preparation Time: 15 min

Cooking Time: 30 min

Mode of Cooking: Baking

Servings: 5

Ingredients:

- 2 sweet potatoes, peeled and cubed
- 3 parsnips, peeled and sliced
- 2 beets, peeled and diced
- 1 red onion, sliced
- 3 Tbsp balsamic vinegar
- 2 Tbsp olive oil
- Salt and freshly ground black pepper to taste
- 1 tsp dried thyme

Directions:

1. Preheat oven to 425°F (220°C)
2. In a large mixing bowl, whisk together balsamic vinegar, olive oil, salt, black pepper, and thyme
3. Add sweet potatoes, parsnips, beets, and red onion, toss to coat evenly
4. Spread the vegetables on a baking sheet in a single layer
5. Roast in the preheated oven until tender and caramelized, about 30 min, stirring halfway through

Tips:

- Try drizzling a little honey over the vegetables before roasting for a touch of sweetness
- Pair with quinoa or a whole grain for a balanced meal

Nutritional Values: Calories: 200, Fat: 7g, Carbs: 33g, Protein: 3g, Sugar: 11g, Sodium: 125mg, Potassium: 516mg, Cholesterol: 0mg

HERB-CRUSTED RACK OF LAMB

Preparation Time: 20 min.

Cooking Time: 30 min.

Mode of Cooking: Roasting

Servings: 4

Ingredients:

- 2 lb. rack of lamb, frenched
- 2 Tbsp. olive oil
- 1 tsp. sea salt
- 1/2 tsp. freshly ground black pepper
- 3 garlic cloves, minced

- 1 Tbsp. fresh rosemary, chopped
- 1 Tbsp. fresh thyme, chopped
- 1 Tbsp. fresh parsley, chopped
- 1/4 cup almond flour

Directions:

1. Preheat oven to 375°F (190°C)
2. Pat the lamb dry and season with salt and pepper
3. Mix olive oil, garlic, rosemary, thyme, and parsley in a bowl
4. Press the herb mixture onto the lamb
5. Coat the herbed lamb with almond flour gently pressing it to adhere
6. Place the lamb on a roasting rack in a roasting pan and roast in the preheated oven until the internal temperature reaches 145°F (for medium-rare), about 30 min.

Tips:

- Let the lamb rest for 10 min. before carving, which ensures the juices redistribute and keep the meat moist
- Serve with a side of roasted vegetables for a complete meal

Nutritional Values: Calories: 410, Fat: 30g, Carbs: 2g, Protein: 35g, Sugar: 0g, Sodium: 650 mg, Potassium: 475 mg, Cholesterol: 105 mg

• 5.3 COMFORTING CLASSICS

FARMHOUSE TURKEY CASSEROLE

Preparation Time: 20 min
Cooking Time: 1 hr
Mode of Cooking: Baking
Servings: 6
Ingredients:

- 2 lb. ground turkey
- 1 large sweet potato, peeled and diced
- 1 cup carrot, diced
- 1 cup celery, diced
- 1 large onion, chopped
- 3 cloves garlic, minced

- 2 Tbsp olive oil
- 1 tsp dried thyme
- 1 tsp dried rosemary
- ½ tsp black pepper
- 1 cup chicken broth, Whole30 compliant
- ¼ cup coconut cream
- 1 Tbsp arrowroot powder mixed with 2 Tbsp water

Directions:

1. Preheat oven to 375°F (190°C)
2. In a large skillet, sauté onions, garlic, carrot, and celery in olive oil until soft
3. Add ground turkey and cook until browned
4. Stir in thyme, rosemary, and black pepper
5. Add sweet potato and chicken broth, bring to a simmer
6. Mix arrowroot powder with water and stir into the skillet to thicken the sauce slightly
7. Transfer mixture to a baking dish
8. Pour coconut cream over the top and bake for 40 min

Tips:

- Use organic vegetables for enhanced flavor and health benefits
- Can be made ahead and refrigerated overnight, flavors enhance with time

Nutritional Values: Calories: 320, Fat: 17g, Carbs: 18g, Protein: 25g, Sugar: 5g, Sodium: 300 mg, Potassium: 600 mg, Cholesterol: 80 mg

SPICED PUMPKIN CHICKEN BAKE

Preparation Time: 15 min
Cooking Time: 45 min
Mode of Cooking: Baking
Servings: 4
Ingredients:

- 4 chicken breasts, boneless and skinless
- 1 can pumpkin puree, no sugar added
- 1 onion, sliced
- 3 cloves garlic, minced
- 1 Tbsp cumin

- 1 tsp cinnamon
- ½ tsp nutmeg
- ½ tsp black pepper
- 2 Tbsp olive oil
- 1 cup chicken broth, Whole30 compliant

Directions:

1. Preheat oven to 400°F (200°C)
2. In a bowl, mix pumpkin puree with garlic, cumin, cinnamon, nutmeg, and black pepper
3. In a skillet, heat olive oil and sauté onions until translucent
4. Place chicken breasts in a baking dish and cover with the pumpkin spice mixture
5. Pour chicken broth around the chicken
6. Bake for 35-40 min or until chicken is cooked through

Tips:

- Serving with a side of roasted vegetables can complement the flavors of the dish
- Cinnamon can be adjusted according to taste preference

Nutritional Values: Calories: 310, Fat: 10g, Carbs: 15g, Protein: 40g, Sugar: 5g, Sodium: 290 mg, Potassium: 800 mg, Cholesterol: 105 mg

LEMON HERB SLOW COOKER PORK

Preparation Time: 10 min

Cooking Time: 8 hr

Mode of Cooking: Slow Cooking

Servings: 6

Ingredients:

- 3 lb. pork shoulder
- 2 lemons, juice and zest
- 1 Tbsp dried oregano
- 1 Tbsp dried basil
- 2 cloves garlic, minced
- 1 onion, chopped
- 1 cup vegetable broth, Whole30 compliant
- Salt to taste
- Pepper to taste
- 2 Tbsp olive oil

Directions:

1. Place the pork shoulder in the slow cooker
2. In a bowl, combine lemon zest, lemon juice, oregano, basil, garlic, salt, and pepper
3. Pour this mixture over the pork
4. Add chopped onion and vegetable broth around the pork
5. Cook on low for 8 hr or until pork is tender and easily shreds with a fork

Tips:

- Pork can be shredded and used in salads or as a filling for lettuce wraps for a lighter meal option
- Adding a splash of apple cider vinegar to the broth brings a nice tangy flavor to the dish

Nutritional Values: Calories: 365, Fat: 20g, Carbs: 8g, Protein: 35g, Sugar: 2g, Sodium: 310 mg, Potassium: 590 mg, Cholesterol: 115 mg

TURKEY AND SWEET POTATO SHEPHERD'S PIE

Preparation Time: 20 min

Cooking Time: 40 min

Mode of Cooking: Baking

Servings: 6

Ingredients:

- 1 lb ground turkey
- 2 large sweet potatoes, peeled and cubed
- 1 Tbsp olive oil
- 1 medium onion, diced
- 2 cloves garlic, minced
- 1 cup carrot, diced
- 1 cup celery, diced
- 2 Tbsp coconut flour
- 1 cup low-sodium chicken broth
- ½ tsp each of dried thyme and rosemary
- Salt and pepper to taste
- 1 Tbsp ghee, melted

Directions:

1. Preheat oven to 400°F (204°C)
2. Boil sweet potatoes until tender, then mash with ghee, salt, and pepper

3. In a skillet, heat olive oil and sauté onion, garlic, carrot, and celery until soft
4. Add ground turkey, cooking until browned
5. Sprinkle coconut flour over meat, stir to coat, then add broth and herbs, simmering until thickened
6. Layer the meat mixture in a baking dish and top with mashed sweet potatoes
7. Bake in the oven for 20 min or until the top is slightly crispy

Tips:

- Toast the coconut flour slightly before adding to enhance flavor.
- Incorporate a pinch of cinnamon to the mashed sweet potatoes for a unique twist
- Adding a dash of paprika for a subtly sweet note

Nutritional Values: Calories: 330, Fat: 15g, Carbs: 28g, Protein: 17g, Sugar: 5g, Sodium: 70 mg, Potassium: 780 mg, Cholesterol: 55 mg

WHOLE30 BEEF STEW

Preparation Time: 15 min
Cooking Time: 8 hr
Mode of Cooking: Slow Cooking
Servings: 8
Ingredients:

- 2 lb chuck beef, cut into cubes
- 3 cup beef broth
- 1 onion, chopped
- 4 carrots, peeled and sliced
- 4 celery stalks, sliced
- 1 bay leaf
- 2 tsp dried parsley
- 2 cloves garlic, minced
- Salt and pepper to taste
- 2 Tbsp tomato paste
- 1 cup turnips, peeled and cubed
- 2 Tbsp olive oil

Directions:

1. Season beef with salt and pepper
2. Heat oil in a skillet and brown the beef over medium heat, then transfer to a slow cooker
3. In the same skillet, add onion, garlic, carrots,and celery, cooking until softened, then transfer to the slow cooker
4. Add all remaining ingredients to the slow cooker, stirring to combine
5. Cover and cook on low for 8 hr or until meat is tender and vegetables are cooked

Tips:

- Deglaze the skillet with some beef broth to capture all the flavorful bits
- Thicken stew by mashing some of the turnips against the side of the slow cooker before serving
- Garnish with fresh parsley for a pop of color and freshness

Nutritional Values: Calories: 350, Fat: 22g, Carbs: 15g, Protein: 25g, Sugar: 5g, Sodium: 200 mg, Potassium: 950 mg, Cholesterol: 80 mg

CHAPTER 6: SNACKING SMART

Picture this: It's mid-afternoon; you've conquered the bulk of your day, but your energy levels are starting to dip. We've all been there, haven't we? The lure of sugary snacks whispers enticingly, promising a quick fix. Yet, deep down, you know they're far from what your body genuinely needs. Herein lies the beauty of smart snacking—a crucial, yet often overlooked, ally in your journey to a wholesome life.

In a world where snack aisles are laden with moreish treats high in refined sugars and artificial additives, the idea of snacking healthily can seem daunting. Yet, the truth is quite the opposite. Embracing whole foods for your snacks can be both a delightful adventure and a profound health catalyst.

Imagine transforming your snacking habit into a source of vitality. Each snack you choose can be a stepping stone towards improved well-being. Whether it's the crunch of fresh veggies dipped in homemade hummus or the soft, sweet bite of a date stuffed with almond butter, smart, whole food snacks effortlessly combine nutrition with convenience.

Moreover, snacking smart isn't just about choosing healthier options; it's about understanding the rhythm of your body's needs. It teaches you to recognize genuine hunger cues, differentiate them from boredom-eating, and select foods that contribute to sustained energy levels. This nuanced approach ensures that each bite you take supports your body's overall nutrition.

This chapter is not just a compilation of recipes. It's a guide to restructuring your snacking ideology, shifting from mindless munching to mindful nourishment. Through a tapestry of tasty and nutritious snacks, we'll explore how these small bites can fit seamlessly into your busy life, an uplifting bridge between meals, keeping you fueled, focused, and on track with your health goals.

So, let's embark on this snacking adventure together, one where every nibble is a treat to your taste buds and a gift to your health. It's time to transform the way we think about snacking, one smart choice at a time.

• 6.1 HEALTHY PLANT-BASED SNACKS

CRISPY KALE CHIPS

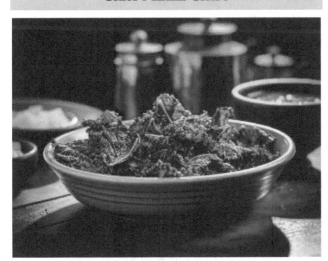

Preparation Time: 10 min
Cooking Time: 15 min
Mode of Cooking: Baking

Servings: 4
Ingredients:

- 1 bunch of kale, stems removed and leaves torn into bite-sized pieces
- 2 Tbsp olive oil
- 1 tsp smoked paprika
- Salt to taste

Directions:

1. Preheat oven to 350°F (175°C)
2. Toss kale pieces with olive oil, smoked paprika, and salt
3. Spread evenly on a baking sheet and bake until crisp, about 15 min, turning halfway through

Tips:

- Store in an airtight container to maintain crispness
- Experiment with different seasonings such as garlic powder or cumin for a new twist

Nutritional Values: Calories: 58, Fat: 4.5g, Carbs: 4.4g, Protein: 2.1g, Sugar: 0.5g, Sodium: 299 mg, Potassium: 213 mg, Cholesterol: 0 mg

SPICED NUT MIX

Preparation Time: 5 min

Cooking Time: 10 min

Mode of Cooking: Roasting

Servings: 6

Ingredients:

- 1 C. raw mixed nuts (almonds, walnuts, pecans)
- 1 Tbsp ghee, melted
- 1 tsp chili powder
- ½ tsp sea salt
- ¼ tsp black pepper
- 1/8 tsp cayenne pepper

Directions:

1. Preheat oven to 350°F (175°C)
2. Combine nuts with melted ghee and spices in a bowl
3. Spread on a baking sheet and roast for 10 min, stirring occasionally

Tips:

- Cool before serving to enhance flavor and crunch
- Nuts can be stored in a cool, dry place for up to 2 weeks

Nutritional Values: Calories: 203, Fat: 18g, Carbs: 7g, Protein: 5g, Sugar: 1g, Sodium: 200 mg, Potassium: 200 mg, Cholesterol: 5 mg

AVOCADO LIME PUDDING

Preparation Time: 10 min

Cooking Time: none

Mode of Cooking: Blending

Servings: 2

Ingredients:

- 1 ripe avocado
- Juice of 1 lime
- 2 Tbsp coconut cream
- 1 Tbsp fresh cilantro, chopped
- 1 tsp lime zest
- Salt and pepper to taste

Directions:

1. Combine all ingredients in a blender and blend until smooth
2. Adjust seasoning with extra lime juice or salt and pepper to taste

Tips:

- This pudding is best enjoyed fresh but can be kept in the fridge for up to 24 hr
- Garnish with extra cilantro or lime zest before serving

Nutritional Values: Calories: 160, Fat: 15g, Carbs: 8g, Protein: 2g, Sugar: 1g, Sodium: 10 mg, Potassium: 485 mg, Cholesterol: 0 mg

SWEET POTATO TOASTS

Preparation Time: 5 min

Cooking Time: 15 min

Mode of Cooking: Baking

Servings: 4

Ingredients:

- 1 large sweet potato, sliced ¼ inch thick
- 2 Tbsp olive oil
- Salt to taste
- Optional toppings: almond butter, banana slices, chia seeds

Directions:

1. Preheat oven to 400°F (200°C)
2. Brush both sides of sweet potato slices with olive oil and season with salt
3. Bake until golden and tender, about 15 min, flipping halfway through

Tips:

● Serve with your choice of toppings like almond butter and banana slices for a sweet option or avocado and radish for a savory one

● Leftover toasts can be refrigerated and reheated in a toaster for quick re-serving

Nutritional Values: Calories: 112, Fat: 7g, Carbs: 12g, Protein: 1g, Sugar: 2g, Sodium: 70 mg, Potassium: 219 mg, Cholesterol: 0 mg

SPICY ROASTED CHICKPEAS

Preparation Time: 10 min

Cooking Time: 40 min

Mode of Cooking: Baking

Servings: 4

Ingredients:

● 1 can chickpeas (15 oz.), drained and rinsed
● 1 Tbsp olive oil
● 1 tsp smoked paprika
● 1 tsp garlic powder
● 1 tsp chili powder
● 1/2 tsp sea salt
● 1/4 tsp black pepper

Directions:

1. Preheat oven to 400°F (200°C)
2. Dry chickpeas thoroughly with a towel
3. In a bowl, toss chickpeas with olive oil and spices until evenly coated
4. Spread chickpeas on a baking sheet in a single layer
5. Bake for 40 min, stirring every 10 min until crispy

Tips:

● Store in an airtight container to maintain crispiness

● Add to salads for extra crunch and flavor

● Adjust spice levels according to taste preference

Nutritional Values: Calories: 134, Fat: 5g, Carbs: 18g, Protein: 6g, Sugar: 0g, Sodium: 300 mg, Potassium: 210 mg, Cholesterol: 0 mg

• 6.2 PROTEIN AND ENERGY BOOSTS

SPICED NUTTY CRUNCH MIX

Preparation Time: 10 min

Cooking Time: 15 min

Mode of Cooking: Baking

Servings: 4

Ingredients:

● 1 C. almonds
● 1 C. pumpkin seeds
● ½ C. sunflower seeds
● 1 Tbsp olive oil
● 1 tsp smoked paprika
● ½ tsp ground cumin
● 1 tsp garlic powder
● ¼ tsp cayenne pepper
● 1 tsp sea salt

Directions:

1. Preheat oven to 350°F (175°C)
2. Combine all nuts and seeds in a bowl
3. In another bowl, mix olive oil with smoked paprika, cumin, garlic powder, cayenne pepper, and sea salt
4. Pour the spice mixture over the nuts and seeds, stir until well coated
5. Spread on a baking sheet and bake for 15 min, stirring halfway through

Tips:

● Store in an airtight container to maintain crispness

● Can be used as a salad topper for extra protein and flavor

Nutritional Values: Calories: 280, Fat: 23g, Carbs: 12g, Protein: 10g, Sugar: 1g, Sodium: 290 mg, Potassium: 300 mg, Cholesterol: 0 mg

TUNA AND AVOCADO ENERGY BALLS

Preparation Time: 15 min

Cooking Time: none

Mode of Cooking: No Cooking

Servings: 8

Ingredients:

- 1 can (5 oz.) tuna, drained
- 1 ripe avocado, peeled and pitted
- ¼ C. red onion, finely chopped
- 1 Tbsp lime juice
- ½ tsp chili flakes
- ¼ C. cilantro, chopped
- Salt and pepper to taste

Directions:

1. Mash the avocado in a bowl
2. Add drained tuna, red onion, lime juice, chili flakes, cilantro, salt, and pepper
3. Mix until well combined
4. Form the mixture into small balls and refrigerate for at least 30 min to firm up

Tips:

- Serve chilled for a refreshing and energizing snack
- Perfect for post-workout or a quick protein boost

Nutritional Values: Calories: 90, Fat: 5g, Carbs: 3g, Protein: 9g, Sugar: 0g, Sodium: 210 mg, Potassium: 180 mg, Cholesterol: 10 mg

BEEF JERKY WITH CITRUS ZEST

Preparation Time: 24 hr
Cooking Time: 4 hr
Mode of Cooking: Drying
Servings: 6
Ingredients:

- 2 lb. lean beef, thinly sliced
- 2 Tbsp coconut aminos
- 1 orange, zest only
- 1 Tbsp black pepper
- 1 tsp sea salt
- ½ tsp chili powder

Directions:

1. Marinate beef slices in coconut aminos, orange zest, black pepper, sea salt, and chili powder for 24 hr

2. Arrange beef on a drying rack over a baking sheet
3. Dry in an oven at 175°F (80°C) for about 4 hr or until fully dehydrated

Tips:

- Use a zip-lock bag for storage to keep jerky fresh longer
- Ideal as a high-protein snack for long hikes or busy days

Nutritional Values: Calories: 250, Fat: 8g, Carbs: 1g, Protein: 40g, Sugar: 0g, Sodium: 590 mg, Potassium: 600 mg, Cholesterol: 90 mg

PUMPKIN-SPICE ENERGY SQUARES

Preparation Time: 15 min
Cooking Time: none
Mode of Cooking: No Cooking
Servings: 12
Ingredients:

- 2 C. rolled oats
- 1 C. pumpkin puree
- ¼ C. flax seeds
- ½ C. pumpkin seeds
- ¼ C. honey (omit for Whole30, use approved sweetener if needed)
- 1 tsp vanilla extract
- 2 tsp pumpkin pie spice
- Pinch of salt

Directions:

1. Combine all ingredients in a large bowl until thoroughly mixed
2. Press the mixture into a lined baking pan
3. Refrigerate for at least 2 hr or until set
4. Cut into squares

Tips:

- Keep refrigerated in an airtight container for up to a week
- Perfect for a quick grab-and-go breakfast or snack

Nutritional Values: Calories: 140, Fat: 5g, Carbs: 20g, Protein: 5g, Sugar: 6g (omit sugar if not using honey), Sodium: 50 mg, Potassium: 135 mg, Cholesterol: 0 mg

SPICED PUMPKIN SEED CRUNCH

Preparation Time: 15 min

Cooking Time: none

Mode of Cooking: No Cooking

Servings: 4

Ingredients:

- 1 cup raw pumpkin seeds
- 1 Tbsp olive oil
- 1 tsp chili powder
- 1 tsp garlic powder
- 1/2 tsp smoked paprika
- 1/2 tsp salt
- 1/4 tsp cayenne pepper

Directions:

1. In a mixing bowl, combine pumpkin seeds and olive oil to coat evenly
2. Sprinkle chili powder, garlic powder, smoked paprika, salt, and cayenne pepper over seeds and stir until well coated
3. Spread evenly on a baking sheet lined with parchment paper
4. Let sit at room temperature to dry for about 1 hr

Tips:

- Store in an airtight container to maintain freshness
- Add to salads or eat solo for a spicy, protein-rich snack

Nutritional Values: Calories: 180, Fat: 15g, Carbs: 4g, Protein: 9g, Sugar: 1g, Sodium: 300 mg, Potassium: 260 mg, Cholesterol: 0 mg

• 6.3 SAVORY TREATS

ROSEMARY ALMOND FLAX CRACKERS

Preparation Time: 15 min

Cooking Time: 20 min

Mode of Cooking: Baking

Servings: 20

Ingredients:

- 2 cups ground flaxseeds
- 1 cup whole almonds, finely chopped
- 2 Tbsp fresh rosemary, chopped
- 1 tsp sea salt
- 1/2 tsp black pepper
- 1/2 cup water

Directions:

1. Combine ground flaxseeds, chopped almonds, rosemary, sea salt, and black pepper in a mixing bowl
2. Gradually add water, stirring until the mixture forms a thick dough
3. Roll out the dough between two sheets of parchment paper to 1/8 inch thickness
4. Remove top parchment and score the dough into squares with a knife
5. Bake in a preheated oven at 350°F (177°C) until crisp and golden, about 20 min
6. Let cool completely and break into squares

Tips:

- Store in an airtight container to maintain crispness
- Pair with a Whole30-compliant dip for added flavor

Nutritional Values: Calories: 130, Fat: 10g, Carbs: 8g, Protein: 5g, Sugar: 0g, Sodium: 120 mg, Potassium: 200 mg, Cholesterol: 0 mg

SPICED COCONUT MEATBALLS

Preparation Time: 25 min

Cooking Time: 15 min

Mode of Cooking: Baking

Servings: 30 meatballs

Ingredients:

- 1 lb ground turkey
- 1/2 cup finely shredded coconut
- 1 Tbsp coconut flour
- 1 egg
- 2 tsp cumin
- 1 tsp smoked paprika
- 1 tsp garlic powder
- 1/2 tsp salt
- 1/4 tsp black pepper

Directions:

1. Mix ground turkey, shredded coconut, coconut flour, egg, cumin, smoked paprika, garlic powder, salt, and pepper in a bowl until well combined
2. Form into small balls and place on a parchment-lined baking sheet
3. Bake in a preheated oven at 375°F (190°C) until golden and cooked through, about 15 min

Tips:

- Serve with a side of mixed greens for a complete snack
- Can be frozen for up to a month for quick snacks

Nutritional Values: Calories: 70, Fat: 4g, Carbs: 2g, Protein: 6g, Sugar: 0g, Sodium: 80 mg, Potassium: 90 mg, Cholesterol: 30 mg

HERB-STUFFED MUSHROOMS

Preparation Time: 10 min

Cooking Time: 25 min

Mode of Cooking: Baking

Servings: 12 mushrooms

Ingredients:

- 12 large mushrooms, stems removed
- 1/4 cup almond meal
- 1/4 cup chopped herbs (parsley, thyme, rosemary)
- 2 cloves garlic, minced
- 1 Tbsp olive oil
- Salt and pepper to taste

Directions:

1. Hollow out the caps of the mushrooms slightly to create space for stuffing
2. Mix almond meal, chopped herbs, minced garlic, olive oil, salt, and pepper in a bowl
3. Stuff the mixture into the mushroom caps
4. Arrange on a baking tray and bake in a preheated oven at 375°F (190°C) for 25 min or until the mushrooms are tender and the topping is golden

Tips:

- Great as a party snack or a light meal
- Leftovers can be reheated for a quick bite

Nutritional Values: Calories: 40, Fat: 3g, Carbs: 2g, Protein: 2g, Sugar: 1g, Sodium: 15 mg, Potassium: 150 mg, Cholesterol: 0 mg

SAVORY PUMPKIN SEEDS

Preparation Time: 5 min

Cooking Time: 15 min

Mode of Cooking: Roasting

Servings: 4

Ingredients:

- 1 cup raw pumpkin seeds
- 1 Tbsp ghee, melted
- 1 tsp chili powder
- 1/2 tsp sea salt
- 1/4 tsp cayenne pepper

Directions:

1. Toss pumpkin seeds with melted ghee, chili powder, sea salt, and cayenne pepper in a bowl
2. Spread evenly on a baking sheet
3. Roast in a preheated oven at 300°F (149°C) for 15 min, stirring occasionally, until toasted and fragrant

Tips:

- A perfect crunchy snack on the go
- Can be sprinkled over salads or soups for extra texture and flavor

Nutritional Values: Calories: 180, Fat: 15g, Carbs: 3g, Protein: 9g, Sugar: 0g, Sodium: 290 mg, Potassium: 260 mg, Cholesterol: 10 mg

SPICY TURMERIC CAULIFLOWER BITES

Preparation Time: 15 min

Cooking Time: 25 min

Mode of Cooking: Baking

Servings: 4

Ingredients:

- 1 head cauliflower, cut into florets
- 2 Tbsp olive oil
- 1 tsp turmeric
- 1 tsp garlic powder
- 1 tsp paprika
- 1/2 tsp cayenne pepper
- Salt and pepper to taste

Directions:

1. Preheat oven to 425°F (220°C)
2. In a large bowl, combine olive oil, turmeric, garlic powder, paprika, cayenne pepper, salt, and pepper
3. Add cauliflower florets and toss to coat evenly
4. Spread on a baking sheet and bake for 25 min, turning halfway through

Tips:

- Serve with a side of homemade Whole30 compliant ranch dressing for dipping
- Store leftovers in an airtight container and reheat for a quick snack

Nutritional Values: Calories: 107, Fat: 7g, Carbs: 10g, Protein: 3g, Sugar: 3g, Sodium: 32mg, Potassium: 320mg, Cholesterol: 0mg

CHAPTER 7: DESSERT TIME

Imagine a world where desserts do more than just satiate your sweet tooth; a world where every bite not only delights your palate but also nourishes your soul and body. Welcome to the sweet, surprising chapter of your healthy eating journey!

Many of us have been conditioned to view desserts as forbidden fruits, packed with unhealthy sugars and fats. However, embarking on a whole food journey doesn't mean you have to turn your back on indulgence and pleasure. In fact, the essence of a sustainable health transformation lies in not just eliminating the harmful, but in enriching your diet with wholesome alternatives that excite and satisfy.

In this chapter, we redefine what it means to treat yourself. Whether you're rounding off a lively family dinner or just need a cozy nightcap that tickles your sweet fancy without the guilt, the recipes here are designed to cater to those desires using fruits, nuts, whole grains, and other unrefined goodies. These ingredients, gifted by nature, are full of the vibrant flavors and nutrients essential for health and happiness.

Consider a velvety chocolate pudding thickened with ripe avocados and sweetened by dates, or a rustic apple crisp topped with a crunchy oat crust, warmly spiced and served right out of the oven. Perhaps the vibrant burst of a lemon tart garnished with fresh raspberries is what tempts you? These desserts are not just treats; they are experiences—wholesome, satisfying, and guilt-free.

Introducing these comforting yet nutritious creations into your routine is like weaving threads of joy into the fabric of everyday life. It's about maintaining balance—indulging your sweet tooth while feeding your well-being. By the end of this chapter, I hope you will feel empowered to create desserts that are not only delectable but also kind to your body, proving that the last course of your meal can indeed be as healthful as it is joyful. Ready to sweeten your days without a pinch of regret? Let's dive in!

• 7.1 FRUIT FAVORITES

TROPICAL MANGO CARPACCIO

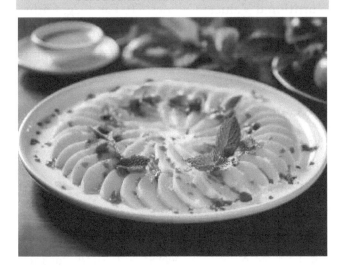

Preparation Time: 10 min
Cooking Time: none
Mode of Cooking: No Cooking
Servings: 4

Ingredients:

- 2 ripe mangoes, peeled and thinly sliced
- 1 small red chili, deseeded and finely chopped
- Zest of 1 lime
- Fresh mint leaves, finely chopped
- 1 Tbsp toasted coconut flakes
- Coconut milk for drizzling

Directions:

1. Arrange mango slices on a serving plate in an overlapping fashion
2. Sprinkle chopped chili, lime zest, and mint over the mangoes
3. Drizzle with coconut milk and garnish with toasted coconut milk

Tips:

- Serve immediately with extra lime wedges for squeezing
- This dish can be personalized by varying the types of chili used for spicing
- Add a dash of sea salt to enhance the flavors

Nutritional Values: Calories: 110, Fat: 2g, Carbs: 25g, Protein: 1g, Sugar: 20g, Sodium: 5 mg, Potassium: 300 mg, Cholesterol: 0 mg

BERRY CITRUS SALAD

Preparation Time: 15 min

Cooking Time: none

Mode of Cooking: No Cooking

Servings: 4

Ingredients:

- 1 cup strawberries, quartered
- 1 cup blueberries
- 2 oranges, peeled and segments cut
- 1 grapefruit, peeled and segments cut
- 2 Tbsp chopped fresh basil
- Drizzle of raw honey (optional, exclude for strict Whole30)
- Juice of 1/2 lemon

Directions:

1. Combine all the fruit in a large bowl
2. Add chopped basil
3. Drizzle with honey if using and lemon juice
4. Toss gently to combine all the flavors

Tips:

- Serve chilled for a refreshing treat
- Can be stored in the refrigerator for up to two days
- Garnish with extra basil before serving to refresh the aroma

Nutritional Values: Calories: 90, Fat: 0.5g, Carbs: 22g, Protein: 1.5g, Sugar: 15g (natural sugars), Sodium: 2 mg, Potassium: 250 mg, Cholesterol: 0 mg

KIWI LIME SORBET

Preparation Time: 15 min

Cooking Time: 2 hr freeze time

Mode of Cooking: Freezing

Servings: 6

Ingredients:

- 6 ripe kiwis, peeled and roughly chopped
- Juice of 3 limes
- 1/4 cup water
- 1 Tbsp honey (optional, exclude for strict Whole30)

Directions:

1. Puree kiwis, lime juice, and water in a blender until smooth
2. Taste and add honey if using
3. Pour into a shallow baking dish and freeze for 2 hours, stirring every 30 minutes

Tips:

- Serve immediately after reaching the desired consistency
- For a creamier texture, process again in a blender before serving
- Garnish with additional lime zest for an extra zing

Nutritional Values: Calories: 70, Fat: 0.2g, Carbs: 17g, Protein: 1g, Sugar: 10g (natural sugars), Sodium: 3 mg, Potassium: 290 mg, Cholesterol: 0 mg

GRILLED PINEAPPLE WITH CINNAMON

Preparation Time: 10 min

Cooking Time: 10 min

Mode of Cooking: Grilling

Servings: 4

Ingredients:

- 1 whole pineapple, peeled and cored, cut into rings
- 1 tsp cinnamon
- 1 Tbsp melted ghee
- Fresh mint for garnish

Directions:

1. Brush pineapple rings with melted ghee and sprinkle with cinnamon
2. Grill on medium heat for about 5 minutes per side or until grill marks appear and pineapple is heated through

Tips:

- Serve warm garnished with fresh mint
- Pineapple can also be cut into wedges if preferred for easier grilling
- Try pairing with coconut yogurt if not following strict Whole30 for a creamy addition

Nutritional Values: Calories: 100, Fat: 3g, Carbs: 19g, Protein: 1g, Sugar: 14g, Sodium: 1 mg, Potassium: 165 mg, Cholesterol: 0 mg

CHILLED MANGO TANGO SLICES

Preparation Time: 15 min

Cooking Time: none

Mode of Cooking: No Cooking

Servings: 4

Ingredients:

- 2 ripe mangos, peeled and thinly sliced
- 1 Tbsp fresh lime juice
- 1 tsp lime zest
- ½ tsp chili powder
- Pinch of sea salt

Directions:

1. Arrange mango slices on a serving plate
2. Drizzle with fresh lime juice and sprinkle with lime zest, chili powder, and sea salt
3. Chill in the refrigerator for 10 minutes before serving

Tips:

- Serve with a sprinkle of fresh mint for an extra zing
- Chili powder can be adjusted according to taste preference

Nutritional Values: Calories: 70, Fat: 0.3g, Carbs: 18g, Protein: 1g, Sugar: 15g, Sodium: 2 mg, Potassium: 168 mg, Cholesterol: 0 mg

---

• 7.2 GUILT-FREE INDULGENCE

AVOCADO LIME MOUSSE

Preparation Time: 15 min

Cooking Time: none

Mode of Cooking: No Cooking

Servings: 4

Ingredients:

- 2 ripe avocados, peeled and pitted
- 1/4 cup fresh lime juice
- Zest of 1 lime
- 1/3 cup coconut cream
- 2 Tbsp raw honey (optional, omit for Whole30)
- 1 tsp pure vanilla extract

Directions:

1. Combine avocados, lime juice, lime zest, coconut cream, honey (if using), and vanilla extract in a food processor
2. Blend until smooth and creamy
3. Transfer to serving dishes and refrigerate for at least 1 hr to set

Tips:

- Opt to chill serving dishes before adding mousse for an extra cool treat
- Garnish with additional lime zest or a sprinkle of sea salt before serving to enhance flavors

Nutritional Values: Calories: 230, Fat: 20g, Carbs: 15g, Protein: 2g, Sugar: 1g, Sodium: 10 mg, Potassium: 487 mg, Cholesterol: 0 mg

COCONUT CACAO NIB BARK

Preparation Time: 10 min

Cooking Time: 1 hr (freezing time)

Mode of Cooking: Freezing

Servings: 8

Ingredients:

- 1 cup coconut butter, melted

- 1/4 cup coconut oil
- 1/4 cup cacao nibs
- 1/4 cup slivered almonds
- 1 tsp cinnamon
- Pinch of sea salt

Directions:

1. Mix melted coconut butter and coconut oil in a bowl
2. Stir in cacao nibs, slivered almonds, cinnamon, and sea salt
3. Pour mixture onto a parchment-lined baking sheet and spread evenly
4. Freeze until solid, about 1 hr
5. Break into pieces

Tips:

- Store in an airtight container in the freezer to keep the bark crisp and fresh
- Sprinkle a tiny amount of coarse sea salt on top before freezing for an enhanced flavor profile

Nutritional Values: Calories: 300, Fat: 29g, Carbs: 8g, Protein: 3g, Sugar: 1g, Sodium: 45 mg, Potassium: 100 mg, Cholesterol: 0 mg

SPICED PEAR SORBET

Preparation Time: 20 min

Cooking Time: 2 hr (freezing time)

Mode of Cooking: Freezing

Servings: 6

Ingredients:

- 4 ripe pears, peeled, cored, and chopped
- 1 Tbsp lemon juice
- 1/4 cup water
- 1 tsp ground cinnamon
- 1/2 tsp ground nutmeg
- 1/2 tsp ground ginger

Directions:

1. Combine pears, lemon juice, water, cinnamon, nutmeg, and ginger in a blender
2. Blend until smooth

3. Pour mixture into a shallow dish and freeze, stirring every 30 min to break up ice crystals, for about 2 hr until firm but scoopable

Tips:

- Serve immediately for best texture
- If sorbet is too hard, let it sit at room temperature for a few minutes before serving
- Experiment with different spices like cardamom or clove for variety

Nutritional Values: Calories: 95, Fat: 0g, Carbs: 25g, Protein: 0g, Sugar: 15g, Sodium: 5 mg, Potassium: 120 mg, Cholesterol: 0 mg

ALMOND BUTTER FUDGE SQUARES

Preparation Time: 15 min

Cooking Time: 2 hr (chilling time)

Mode of Cooking: Chilling

Servings: 12

Ingredients:

- 1 cup almond butter
- 1/2 cup coconut oil, softened
- 1/4 cup unsweetened shredded coconut
- 2 Tbsp raw honey (optional, omit for Whole30)
- 1/2 tsp vanilla extract
- Pinch of sea salt

Directions:

1. Mix almond butter, coconut oil, shredded coconut, honey (if using), vanilla extract, and sea salt until well combined
2. Pour mixture into a lined 8x8 inch square baking dish
3. Refrigerate until set, about 2 hr
4. Cut into squares

Tips:

- Use crunchy almond butter for added texture
- Store in refrigerator to maintain firmness
- Drizzle with melted unsweetened chocolate after chilling for a decadent touch, if desired

Nutritional Values: Calories: 200, Fat: 18g, Carbs: 6g, Protein: 4g, Sugar: 2g, Sodium: 40 mg, Potassium: 200 mg, Cholesterol: 0 mg

AVOCADO CHOCOLATE MOUSSE

Preparation Time: 15 min
Cooking Time: none
Mode of Cooking: No Cooking
Servings: 4
Ingredients:

- 2 ripe avocados, peeled and pitted
- 1/4 C. cocoa powder, unsweetened
- 1/4 C. coconut cream
- 1 tsp vanilla extract
- pinch of salt
- optional erythritol or stevia to taste

Directions:

1. Blend avocados, cocoa powder, coconut cream, vanilla extract, and salt in a food processor until smooth
2. If desired, sweeten to taste with erythritol or stevia
3. Spoon into serving dishes and chill until ready to serve

Tips:

- Using well-ripened avocados will enhance the creaminess without the need for dairy
- Sprinkle with unsweetened shredded coconut for a decorative touch and additional flavor

Nutritional Values: Calories: 200, Fat: 15g, Carbs: 17g, Protein: 2g, Sugar: 1g, Sodium: 10 mg, Potassium: 487 mg, Cholesterol: 0 mg

• 7.3 COZY DESSERTS

WARM SPICED APPLE CRUMBLE

Preparation Time: 20 min
Cooking Time: 35 min
Mode of Cooking: Baking
Servings: 6

Ingredients:

- 3 large apples, peeled and sliced
- 1 Tbsp fresh lemon juice
- 1 tsp ground cinnamon
- ½ tsp ground nutmeg
- ¼ cup almond flour
- ⅓ cup chopped walnuts
- 2 Tbsp coconut oil, melted
- 1 Tbsp flaxseed meal
- 1 tsp vanilla extract
- Pinch of salt

Directions:

1. Preheat oven to 350°F (175°C)
2. Toss apples with lemon juice, cinnamon, and nutmeg and spread in a baking dish
3. Combine almond flour, walnuts, melted coconut oil, flaxseed meal, vanilla extract, and salt in a bowl until mixture is crumbly
4. Sprinkle crumble mixture over the apples
5. Bake until apples are tender and topping is golden brown, about 35 min

Tips:

- Serve warm with a dollop of coconut cream for added delight
- Store leftovers in an airtight container in the refrigerator
- Reheat in the oven for best results

Nutritional Values: Calories: 200, Fat: 11g, Carbs: 24g, Protein: 2g, Sugar: 16g, Sodium: 10 mg, Potassium: 134 mg, Cholesterol: 0 mg

CHAI-SPICED COCONUT CUSTARD

Preparation Time: 10 min
Cooking Time: 40 min
Mode of Cooking: Baking
Servings: 4
Ingredients:

- 1 can full-fat coconut milk
- 4 large eggs
- 2 Tbsp erythritol
- 1 tsp ground cinnamon

- ½ tsp ground cardamom
- ¼ tsp ground cloves
- ¼ tsp ground ginger
- Pinch of salt
- Unsweetened shredded coconut for topping

Directions:

1. Preheat oven to 325°F (163°C)
2. Whisk together coconut milk, eggs, erythritol, cinnamon, cardamom, cloves, ginger, and salt
3. Pour mixture into ramekins
4. Place ramekins in a baking dish and pour hot water into the dish until halfway up the sides of the ramekins
5. Bake until custard is set, about 40 min

Tips:

- Sprinkle with unsweetened shredded coconut before serving
- Can be served warm or chilled
- Garnish with a cinnamon stick for a festive touch

Nutritional Values: Calories: 270, Fat: 21g, Carbs: 8g, Protein: 6g, Sugar: 2g, Sodium: 70 mg, Potassium: 200 mg, Cholesterol: 186 mg

CINNAMON ROASTED PEARS WITH PECAN CRUNCH

Preparation Time: 15 min
Cooking Time: 25 min
Mode of Cooking: Baking
Servings: 4
Ingredients:

- 4 ripe but firm pears, halved and cored
- 2 Tbsp coconut oil, melted
- 2 Tbsp honey (omit for strict Whole30, substitute with a dash of additional cinnamon)
- 1 tsp ground cinnamon
- ¼ cup chopped pecans
- Pinch of salt

Directions:

1. Preheat oven to 375°F (190°C)
2. Arrange pear halves cut side up on a baking sheet
3. Drizzle with melted coconut oil and honey (if using), then sprinkle with cinnamon
4. Roast until pears are tender, about 25 min
5. Sprinkle with chopped pecans and roast for another 5 min

Tips:

- Perfect paired with a sprinkle of nutmeg or served with a side of whipped coconut cream
- Pears can be prepped ahead and roasted just before serving
- Choose pears that are just ripe to avoid mushiness when roasting

Nutritional Values: Calories: 210, Fat: 11g, Carbs: 31g, Protein: 1g, Sugar: 20g (less if omitting honey), Sodium: 5 mg, Potassium: 150 mg, Cholesterol: 0 mg

GINGER PUMPKIN MOUSSE

Preparation Time: 15 min
Cooking Time: none
Mode of Cooking: Mixing
Servings: 6
Ingredients:

- 1 can pumpkin puree
- 1 can full-fat coconut milk, chilled overnight
- 3 Tbsp real maple syrup (omit for strict Whole30, substitute with juice of 1 orange)
- 1 tsp vanilla extract
- 2 tsp ground ginger
- ½ tsp ground cinnamon
- ¼ tsp ground nutmeg
- Pinch of salt

Directions:

1. Combine chilled coconut milk (only the thick cream from the top of the can), pumpkin puree, maple syrup (or orange juice), vanilla

extract, ginger, cinnamon, nutmeg, and salt in a large bowl

2. Use an electric mixer to beat until fluffy and smooth

Tips:

● This dessert is lighter when served immediately but can also be chilled for a couple of hours to firm up

● Top with a sprinkle of cinnamon or coconut flakes for extra texture and flavor

● Great as a festive dessert for fall gatherings

Nutritional Values: Calories: 120, Fat: 7g, Carbs: 13g, Protein: 2g, Sugar: 8g (less if substituting orange juice), Sodium: 20 mg, Potassium: 90 mg, Cholesterol: 0 mg

BAKED CINNAMON APPLE CRISPS

Preparation Time: 15 min

Cooking Time: 2 hr

Mode of Cooking: Baking

Servings: 4

Ingredients:

● 2 large apples, thinly sliced

● 1 Tbsp ground cinnamon

● 1 Tbsp coconut oil, melted

Directions:

1. Preheat oven to 225°F (107°C)
2. Toss apple slices with melted coconut oil and cinnamon until well coated
3. Arrange slices in a single layer on a baking sheet lined with parchment paper
4. Bake in the oven for 2 hours, flipping halfway through until the apple slices are dried and crisp

Tips:

● Store in an airtight container to maintain crispness

● Experiment with other spices like nutmeg or clove for variety

Nutritional Values: Calories: 95, Fat: 3.5g, Carbs: 17g, Protein: 0.5g, Sugar: 12g, Sodium: 2 mg, Potassium: 195 mg, Cholesterol: 0 mg

CHAPTER 8: REFRESHING BEVERAGES

Imagine this: you've just enjoyed a wholesome, fulfilling meal from our earlier chapters, your taste buds are satisfied, but there's still something missing—perhaps a touch of sweetness or a zesty zing to perfectly round out the dining experience. Enter our refreshing beverages—a vibrant chapter dedicated to invigorating drinks, each brimming with health benefits and flavors that cleanse, energize, and soothe.

In the journey of revitalizing your diet, hydration plays a crucial role, often overshadowed by the focus on solids. Here, we elevate beverages to an art form, treating them as integral components of your wellness routine. From the morning rush to the calming close of day, these drinks are crafted to accompany every moment with a splash of nourishment.

Think of your kitchen as a mini alchemist's lab, where ingredients like fresh, plump berries, crisp cucumbers, and vibrant herbs are transformed into more than just refreshments; they become elixirs of health. Each recipe in this chapter is designed to be as delightful to the senses as they are beneficial to the body. Whether it's a smoothie packed with antioxidants, a herbal tea that promises tranquility, or a warm, spicy tonic that fires up your metabolism, these beverages are your daily partners in hydration and health.

Let's not forget the social magic these drinks can weave. Picture hosting a gathering where your guests are not only impressed by the flavors but also leave feeling rejuvenated treated. These creations are not just drinks but conversation starters and mood enhancers.

So, grab your favorite glass and prepare to fill it with more than just a drink. Fill it with vibrant nutrition, with colors that dazzle, tastes that thrill, and aromas that transport you. Whether it's a chilly morning or a warm evening, you will find the perfect beverage here to elevate your day and sustain your journey towards a lasting whole food lifestyle.

• 8.1 ENERGIZING DRINKS

GREEN GINGER ZING SMOOTHIE

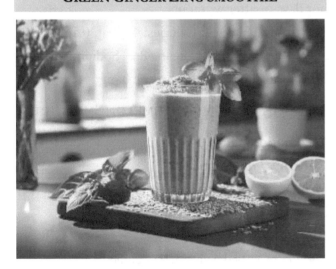

Preparation Time: 10 min.
Cooking Time: none
Mode of Cooking: Blending
Servings: 2

Ingredients:

- 1 ripe avocado, peeled and pitted
- 1 medium cucumber, sliced
- 2 cups fresh spinach leaves
- 1 small piece of ginger, peeled and minced (about 1 tbsp)
- 1 tbsp chia seeds
- 2 cups cold water
- Juice of 1 lime
- Fresh mint leaves for garnish

Directions:

1. Combine avocado, cucumber, spinach, ginger, chia seeds, water, and lime juice in a blender
2. Blend on high until smooth and creamy

3. Pour into glasses and garnish with mint leaves

Tips:

- Add a scoop of plant-based protein powder for a protein boost
- If the smoothie is too thick, adjust the consistency by adding more water
- For extra zest, add a pinch of cayenne pepper

Nutritional Values: Calories: 184, Fat: 12g, Carbs: 17g, Protein: 4g, Sugar: 2g, Sodium: 32 mg, Potassium: 708 mg, Cholesterol: 0 mg

CARROT BEET BLISS JUICE

Preparation Time: 15 min.

Cooking Time: none

Mode of Cooking: Juicing

Servings: 2

Ingredients:

- 4 large carrots, peeled
- 2 medium beets, peeled and quartered
- 1 apple, cored and sliced
- 1-inch piece of turmeric root, peeled
- 1 lemon, peeled and quartered

Directions:

1. Run carrots, beets, apple, turmeric root, and lemon through a juicer
2. Stir to combine and pour over ice if desired
3. Serve immediately

Tips:

- Juice ginger instead of turmeric for a different flavor profile
- Store any leftover juice in a tightly sealed container in the refrigerator and consume within 24 hours
- Consuming this juice in the morning may provide an energizing start to the day

Nutritional Values: Calories: 95, Fat: 0.3g, Carbs: 22g, Protein: 2g, Sugar: 14g, Sodium: 76 mg, Potassium: 687 mg, Cholesterol: 0 mg

SPICY PINEAPPLE CUCUMBER WATER

Preparation Time: 10 min.

Cooking Time: none

Mode of Cooking: Mixing

Servings: 4

Ingredients:

- ½ pineapple, peeled and cubed
- 1 large cucumber, sliced
- 1 small jalapeño, seeded and thinly sliced
- 8 cups cold water
- Juice of 2 limes
- Fresh cilantro leaves for garnish

Directions:

1. In a large pitcher, combine pineapple, cucumber, jalapeño, and water
2. Stir in lime juice
3. Refrigerate for at least 2 hours to allow the flavors to meld
4. Serve chilled, garnished with cilantro leaves

Tips:

- For a sweeter drink, add a little stevia or honey
- Remove the jalapeño slices after refrigerating if you prefer a milder flavor
- This refreshing water is ideal for hydration on hot days or after workouts

Nutritional Values: Calories: 46, Fat: 0.1g, Carbs: 12g, Protein: 0.5g, Sugar: 8g, Sodium: 5 mg, Potassium: 120 mg, Cholesterol: 0 mg

COOLING MINTY WATERMELON SMOOTHIE

Preparation Time: 10 min.

Cooking Time: none

Mode of Cooking: Blending

Servings: 2

Ingredients:

- 2 cups cubed watermelon, chilled
- ½ cup fresh mint leaves
- Juice of 1 lime
- 1 cup coconut water
- Ice cubes (optional)

- 1 tbsp flax seeds

Directions:

1. Place watermelon, mint leaves, lime juice, coconut water, ice cubes (if using), and flax seeds in a blender
2. Blend until smooth
3. Pour into glasses and serve immediately

Tips:

- Add a pinch of salt to enhance the sweetness of the watermelon
- For an extra chill factor, freeze the cubed watermelon prior to blending
- Garnish with extra mint leaves for a decorative touch

Nutritional Values: Calories: 71, Fat: 1.2g, Carbs: 14g, Protein: 1.6g, Sugar: 10g, Sodium: 42 mg, Potassium: 270 mg, Cholesterol: 0 mg

COCONUT WATER REFRESHER

Preparation Time: 3 min.

Cooking Time: none

Mode of Cooking: Mixing

Servings: 1

Ingredients:

- 1 C. coconut water
- 1/2 C. fresh pineapple chunks
- 1/3 C. mango chunks
- 1/2 lime, juiced
- A few mint leaves
- Ice cubes

Directions:

1. Pour coconut water into a blender
2. Add pineapple chunks, mango chunks, and lime juice
3. Blend until smooth
4. Serve over ice and garnish with mint leaves

Tips:

- This drink is hydrating and perfect for post-workout recovery

- Mint is not only for flavor but also aids in digestion

Nutritional Values: Calories: 75, Fat: 0.2g, Carbs: 18g, Protein: 1g, Sugar: 15g, Sodium: 25mg, Potassium: 500mg, Cholesterol: 0mg

• 8.2 TEAS AND INFUSIONS

LAVENDER AND CHAMOMILE INFUSION

Preparation Time: 5 min

Cooking Time: 10 min

Mode of Cooking: Steeping

Servings: 2

Ingredients:

- 2 Tbsp dried lavender flowers
- 2 Tbsp dried chamomile flowers
- 4 cups boiling water
- 1 tsp raw honey (optional, if off Whole30)
- 1 lemon slice for garnish

Directions:

1. Combine lavender and chamomile flowers in a teapot
2. Pour boiling water over the flowers and let steep for 10 minutes
3. Strain the infusion into cups and sweeten with honey if desired, garnish with a lemon slice

Tips:

- Serve warm for a relaxing evening drink, especially beneficial before bedtime
- Add a fresh mint leaf for a refreshing twist
- To preserve the delicate flavors, do not overheat the water

Nutritional Values: Calories: 2, Fat: 0g, Carbs: 0.5g, Protein: 0g, Sugar: 0g (without honey), Sodium: 2 mg, Potassium: 9 mg, Cholesterol: 0 mg

GINGER TURMERIC BONE BROTH

Preparation Time: 10 min

Cooking Time: 4 hr

Mode of Cooking: Simmering

Servings: 6

Ingredients:

- 4 cups beef bone broth (Whole30 compliant)
- 1 inch fresh turmeric root, grated
- 1 inch fresh ginger root, grated
- 1 garlic clove, minced
- pinch of black pepper
- 1 Tbsp apple cider vinegar
- 1 green onion, chopped for garnish

Directions:

1. Combine all ingredients except green onion in a large pot
2. Bring to a simmer and maintain it for 4 hours on low heat, occasionally skimming the surface
3. Strain broth through a fine sieve, garnish with green onion

Tips:

- Drink hot to maximize digestion-enhancing properties
- Can be stored in the refrigerator for up to 5 days or frozen for future use
- Stir well before re-heating as spices might settle at the bottom

Nutritional Values: Calories: 40, Fat: 0.5g, Carbs: 2g, Protein: 6g, Sugar: 0g, Sodium: 120 mg, Potassium: 370 mg, Cholesterol: 0 mg

REFRESHING MINT AND LEMON BALM TEA

Preparation Time: 5 min

Cooking Time: 5 min

Mode of Cooking: Steeping

Servings: 4

Ingredients:

- 2 Tbsp fresh mint leaves
- 2 Tbsp fresh lemon balm leaves
- 4 cups boiling water
- lemon slices for garnish

Directions:

1. Place mint and lemon balm leaves in a large teapot
2. Cover with boiling water and let steep for 5 minutes
3. Strain the tea into cups and add a lemon slice in each

Tips:

- Use freshly picked herbs for the most potent flavor
- Refrigerate any leftovers and enjoy cold for a revitalizing drink
- Crush the leaves gently with your fingers before adding boiling water to release more essential oils

Nutritional Values: Calories: 0, Fat: 0g, Carbs: 0g, Protein: 0g, Sugar: 0g, Sodium: 1 mg, Potassium: 12 mg, Cholesterol: 0 mg

SOOTHING CINNAMON AND STAR ANISE INFUSION

Preparation Time: 5 min

Cooking Time: 15 min

Mode of Cooking: Steeping

Servings: 3

Ingredients:

- 3 star anise pods
- 1 cinnamon stick
- 4 cups water
- 2 cardamom pods, crushed

Directions:

1. Combine star anise pods, cinnamon stick, cardamom pods, and water in a saucepan
2. Bring to a boil then reduce to a simmer for 15 minutes
3. Strain the infusion into mugs

Tips:

- Ideal for a calming evening beverage
- Add a splash of coconut milk for a creamy texture and extra layer of flavor

● For a sweeter taste, add a drop of stevia (if not on Whole30)

Nutritional Values: Calories: 2, Fat: 0g, Carbs: 1g, Protein: 0g, Sugar: 0g, Sodium: 5 mg, Potassium: 10 mg, Cholesterol: 0 mg

LEMONGRASS GINGER INFUSION

Preparation Time: 5 min
Cooking Time: 15 min
Mode of Cooking: Simmering
Servings: 2
Ingredients:
● 2 stalks fresh lemongrass, crushed
● 1 inch fresh ginger root, sliced
● 4 cups water
● 1 Tbsp honey (optional for non-Whole30 compliance)
● 1 tsp fresh lemon juice

Directions:

1. Bring water to a boil in a saucepan
2. Add crushed lemongrass and sliced ginger
3. Reduce heat and simmer for 15 min
4. Remove from heat and stir in lemon juice
5. Strain into cups and sweeten with honey if desired

Tips:

● Enjoy hot or chilled over ice for a refreshing twist

● To enhance flavor, let the infusion steep overnight in the refrigerator

Nutritional Values: Calories: 9, Fat: 0g, Carbs: 2g, Protein: 0g, Sugar: 1g (excluding optional honey), Sodium: 1 mg, Potassium: 10 mg, Cholesterol: 0 mg

• 8.3 WARM AND INVITING

SPICED GOLDEN MILK

Preparation Time: 5 min
Cooking Time: 10 min
Mode of Cooking: Simmer
Servings: 2

Ingredients:
● 2 cups of almond milk
● 1 Tbsp grated fresh turmeric
● 1 tsp grated fresh ginger
● 1 cinnamon stick
● 1 Tbsp coconut oil
● 1 pinch of black pepper
● 1 tsp honey (optional, omit for Whole30 compliance)

Directions:

1. Combine almond milk, turmeric, ginger, and cinnamon stick in a saucepan and bring to a simmer over medium heat
2. Simmer for 10 min, then remove from heat and stir in coconut butter and black pepper
3. Strain the mixture into mugs

Tips:

● Serve warm and stir well before drinking to mix the oil thoroughly into the milk

● Add a cinnamon stick for garnish if desired

● If not following Whole30, a teaspoon of honey can add a lovely sweetness

Nutritional Values: Calories: 120, Fat: 11g, Carbs: 4g, Protein: 1g, Sugar: 0g (1g if honey is added), Sodium: 120 mg, Potassium: 50 mg, Cholesterol: 0 mg

HERBAL LAVENDER TEA

Preparation Time: 2 min
Cooking Time: 5 min
Mode of Cooking: Steep
Servings: 2
Ingredients:
● 2 cups of water
● 1 Tbsp dried lavender flowers
● 1 tsp dried chamomile
● 1 tsp honey (optional, omit for Whole30 compliance)
● slices of lemon for serving

Directions:

1. Bring water to a boil
2. Add lavender and chamomile to the boiling water and remove from heat
3. Cover and let steep for 5 min
4. Strain into teacups and add a slice of lemon to each cup

Tips:

- This tea is perfect for relaxation before bedtime
- Can be enjoyed cold as well by allowing it to cool and refrigerating for an hour

Nutritional Values: Calories: 0, Fat: 0g, Carbs: 0g (1g if honey is added), Protein: 0g, Sugar: 0g (1g if honey is added), Sodium: 0 mg, Potassium: 9 mg, Cholesterol: 0 mg

CINNAMON COCONUT HOT CHOCOLATE

Preparation Time: 5 min

Cooking Time: 5 min

Mode of Cooking: Mix and Heat

Servings: 2

Ingredients:

- 2 cups of coconut milk
- 2 Tbsp cocoa powder
- ½ tsp ground cinnamon
- 1 Tbsp almond butter
- 1 pinch of sea salt
- 1 tsp vanilla extract

Directions:

1. Heat coconut milk in a saucepan over medium heat until hot but not boiling
2. Whisk in cocoa powder, cinnamon, almond butter, sea salt, and vanilla extract until smooth and creamy

Tips:

- Top with a sprinkle of cinnamon or coconut flakes for extra flavor and presentation
- Great as a comforting drink during chilly evenings

Nutritional Values: Calories: 150, Fat: 12g, Carbs: 8g, Protein: 3g, Sugar: 2g, Sodium: 150 mg, Potassium: 200 mg, Cholesterol: 0 mg

WARM GINGER LEMONADE

Preparation Time: 10 min

Cooking Time: 5 min

Mode of Cooking: Simmer

Servings: 2

Ingredients:

- 2 cups of water
- 1 inch fresh ginger, sliced
- Juice of 2 lemons
- 1 tsp honey (optional, omit for Whole30 compliance)

Directions:

1. Combine water and ginger slices in a pot and bring to a boil
2. Simmer for 10 min to infuse the ginger flavor
3. Remove from heat and stir in lemon juice
4. Strain into mugs

Tips:

- Can be served with a slice of lemon or a sprig of mint for a fresh touch
- Honey can be added for sweetness if not following Whole30.

Nutritional Values: Calories: 10, Fat: 0g, Carbs: 3g, Protein: 0g, Sugar: 0g (1g if honey is added), Sodium: 10 mg, Potassium: 30 mg, Cholesterol: 0 mg

GOLDEN TURMERIC MILK

Preparation Time: 5 min.

Cooking Time: 10 min.

Mode of Cooking: Stovetop

Servings: 2

Ingredients:

- 1½ cups of unsweetened almond milk
- 1 tsp of turmeric powder
- ¼ tsp ground cinnamon

- 1/8 tsp ground ginger
- Pinch of black pepper
- 1 tsp of coconut oil
- 1 tsp of date paste for sweetness

Directions:

1. Combine almond milk, turmeric, cinnamon, ginger, and black pepper in a small saucepan and heat over medium heat until just simmering
2. Add coconut oil and date paste, and whisk until fully integrated and the mixture is heated through
3. Remove from heat and pour into mugs

Tips:

- Add a cinnamon stick for stirring and extra flavor
- Serve warm to maximize the soothing effects

Nutritional Values: Calories: 60, Fat: 4.5g, Carbs: 5g, Protein: 1g, Sugar: 4g, Sodium: 120 mg, Potassium: 50 mg, Cholesterol: 0 mg

CHAPTER 9: FAMILY-FRIENDLY MEALS

When envisioning a family-friendly meal, what often comes to mind are relaxed, giggly evenings filled with nutritious foods that not only appease your health goals but also win the hearts of the tiny critics at your table. In many homes, mealtime is an oasis—a precious window where stories and smiles are exchanged over plates of wholesome food. However, as harmonious as this sounds, the reality of preparing meals that everyone from toddlers to teens will enjoy can sometimes feel like navigating a culinary obstacle course.

In this chapter, I aim to arm you with a treasure trove of recipes that bridge the gap between nutritious and delightful, ensuring your kitchen becomes a source of health and happiness without stress. Think of dishes that invoke a sense of comfort yet are packed with the goodness of whole foods—meals that are crafted cleverly to be both enticing and enriching.

Imagine the scene: it's a weekday evening, and instead of the usual hustle to cobble together a meal that meets everyone's approval, you find yourself smiling as you prepare a one-pan dish that's bursting with colors and flavors. Kids are curious, poking their heads around the corner, enticed by the familiar yet intriguing aromas wafting through your home. These recipes aren't just meant to be eaten; they're meant to be explored and enjoyed, forming part of the stories that your family will cherish.

Not only will these meals help foster a love for whole foods among the younger members of your household, but they will also ease the often-exhausting dilemma of balancing a busy schedule with the desire to provide nourishing meals. From breakfasts that can be whipped up in a flash yet power them through their morning, to lunches that are perfect for piling into a box, and dinners that turn into family favorites, each recipe is a step towards making whole food a joyful and permanent resident in your family's life. Let's embrace the challenge and delight of feeding our families, transforming necessity into an enjoyable journey for everyone involved.

• 9.1 KID-FRIENDLY BREAKFASTS

BANANA ALMOND BUTTER PANCAKES

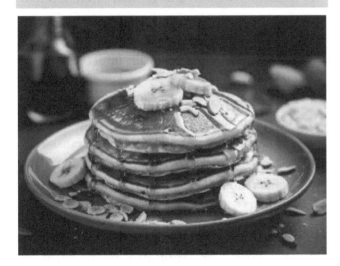

Preparation Time: 15 min
Cooking Time: 10 min
Mode of Cooking: Pan Frying
Servings: 4

Ingredients:

- 2 ripe bananas, mashed
- 1 cup almond flour
- 3 large eggs
- 1/4 cup almond butter
- 1/2 tsp baking soda
- 1/2 tsp cinnamon
- 1 Tbsp coconut oil for cooking

Directions:

1. Mash bananas in a mixing bowl
2. Add almond flour, eggs, almond butter, baking soda, and cinnamon to the bowl and mix until well combined
3. Heat coconut oil in a skillet over medium heat
4. Pour 1/4 cup of batter for each pancake into the skillet

5. Cook for about 3-4 min on each side or until pancakes are golden brown and cooked through

Tips:

• Serve with fresh fruit slices for added sweetness and nutrition

• Ensure pancakes are thoroughly cooked by maintaining a consistent heat

• Encourage kids to help with mashing bananas to make this a fun family activity

Nutritional Values: Calories: 280, Fat: 18g, Carbs: 22g, Protein: 12g, Sugar: 12g, Sodium: 150 mg, Potassium: 300 mg, Cholesterol: 150 mg

MORNING RAINBOW VEGGIE EGG MUFFINS

Preparation Time: 20 min
Cooking Time: 25 min
Mode of Cooking: Baking
Servings: 12
Ingredients:

• 8 large eggs
• 1/2 cup diced red bell pepper
• 1/2 cup diced green bell pepper
• 1/2 cup diced yellow bell pepper
• 1/4 cup diced onion
• 1/4 cup chopped spinach
• 1 tsp garlic powder
• Salt and black pepper to taste
• 1 Tbsp olive oil

Directions:

1. Whisk eggs in a large bowl
2. Add all diced veggies, chopped spinach, garlic powder, salt, and black and stir to combine
3. Grease a 12-cup muffin tin with olive oil
4. Pour the egg mixture into the muffin cups, filling each about 2/3 full
5. Bake in a preheated oven at 350°F (175°C) for 25 min or until the egg muffins are set and edges are slightly golden

Tips:

• These egg muffins can be made in advance for a quick breakfast option throughout the week

• Get creative with veggies according to what your child loves or seasonal availability

Nutritional Values: Calories: 90, Fat: 6g, Carbs: 2g, Protein: 6g, Sugar: 1g, Sodium: 80 mg, Potassium: 120 mg, Cholesterol: 140 mg

SWEET POTATO AND CHICKEN APPLE SAUSAGE HASH

Preparation Time: 15 min
Cooking Time: 20 min
Mode of Cooking: Sautéing
Servings: 4
Ingredients:

• 2 medium sweet potatoes, peeled and diced
• 1 lb chicken apple sausage, sliced
• 1 medium onion, diced
• 1/2 cup green onions, sliced
• 1/4 tsp smoked paprika
• Salt and black pepper to taste
• 2 Tbsp olive oil

Directions:

1. Heat olive oil in a large skillet over medium heat
2. Add diced sweet potatoes and cook for about 10 min, stirring occasionally until they start to soften
3. Add the sliced sausage and diced onion to the skillet and cook for another 10 min until the sausage is browned and onions are translucent
4. Season with smoked paprika, salt, and black pepper, and stir in sliced green onions before serving

Tips:

• This hearty breakfast can be prepared in advance and reheated for busy mornings

• Engage children by letting them help with peeling and dicing the sweet potatoes

Nutritional Values: Calories: 320, Fat: 18g, Carbs: 24g, Protein: 14g, Sugar: 7g, Sodium: 690 mg, Potassium: 530 mg, Cholesterol: 60 mg

COCONUT YOGURT PARFAIT WITH MIXED BERRIES AND NUTS

Preparation Time: 10 min
Cooking Time: none
Mode of Cooking: No Cooking
Servings: 4
Ingredients:

- 2 cups unsweetened coconut yogurt
- 1 cup fresh blueberries
- 1 cup fresh raspberries
- 1/2 cup chopped walnuts
- 1 Tbsp chia seeds
- 1 tsp vanilla extract

Directions:

1. In four serving glasses, layer coconut yogurt, fresh blueberries, raspberries, and chopped walnuts
2. Sprinkle chia seeds and a drizzle of vanilla extract on top of each parfait before serving

Tips:

- Perfect for a quick, no-cook breakfast or a nutritious snack
- Involve kids by letting them choose their favorite berries or nuts to customize their parfaits

Nutritional Values: Calories: 240, Fat: 18g, Carbs: 16g, Protein: 4g, Sugar: 8g, Sodium: 15 mg, Potassium: 180 mg, Cholesterol: 0 mg

BANANA ALMOND PANCAKES

Preparation Time: 10 min.
Cooking Time: 8 min.
Mode of Cooking: Pan frying
Servings: 4
Ingredients:

- 2 ripe bananas, mashed
- 1 cup almond flour

- 2 large eggs
- 1/2 tsp baking soda
- 1/4 tsp salt
- 1/2 tsp cinnamon
- 1 tsp vanilla extract
- Ghee for frying

Directions:

1. Mash bananas in a mixing bowl
2. Add eggs and vanilla, blend thoroughly
3. Combine almond flour, baking soda, salt, and cinnamon in another bowl
4. Mix dry ingredients with wet ingredients to form batter
5. Heat ghee in a skillet over medium heat
6. Pour 1/4 cup of batter for each pancake
7. Cook until bubbles form on top, then flip and cook until browned

Tips:

- Serve with a sprinkle of cinnamon and fresh banana slices for extra sweetness without the added sugar
- For a nuttier flavor, add a small handful of chopped almonds into the batter before cooking
- Always use ripe bananas for natural sweetness and better binding

Nutritional Values: Calories: 280, Fat: 18g, Carbs: 23g, Protein: 9g, Sugar: 7g, Sodium: 400 mg, Potassium: 300 mg, Cholesterol: 93 mg

---

• 9.2 LUNCHBOX CREATIONS

TURKEY AND VEGGIE COLLAGE WRAP

Preparation Time: 15 min
Cooking Time: none
Mode of Cooking: No Cooking
Servings: 4
Ingredients:

- 4 large collard green leaves, blanched
- 8 oz. turkey breast, thinly sliced
- 1 carrot, julienned
- 1 red bell pepper, julienned

- 1 cucumber, julienned
- 1 small avocado, sliced
- 2 Tbsp homemade paleo mayonnaise
- Fresh cilantro, chopped

Directions:

1. Lay out blanched collard greens on a flat surface
2. Spread a thin layer of paleo mayonnaise over each leaf
3. Layer turkey slices and julienned vegetables on one edge of each leaf
4. Add slices of avocado and sprinkle with cilantro
5. Roll up tightly, starting from the edge with the fillings, and cut into pinwheels

Tips:

- Serve with a side of mixed berries for a fruity touch
- Can be prepared the night before and kept in a cool place until lunch

Nutritional Values: Calories: 250, Fat: 9g, Carbs: 12g, Protein: 25g, Sugar: 3g, Sodium: 300 mg, Potassium: 400 mg, Cholesterol: 50 mg

SWEET POTATO CHICKEN NUGGETS

Preparation Time: 30 min
Cooking Time: 20 min
Mode of Cooking: Baking
Servings: 4
Ingredients:

- 1 lb. ground chicken
- 1 medium sweet potato, cooked and mashed
- 1 tsp garlic powder
- 1 tsp onion powder
- 1 Tbsp coconut flour
- Salt and pepper to taste
- Olive oil for greasing

Directions:

1. Preheat oven to 375°F (190°C)

2. In a large bowl, combine ground chicken with mashed sweet potato, garlic powder, onion powder, coconut flour, salt, and pepper
3. Mix well until all ingredients are thoroughly combined
4. Form into small, flat nuggets and place on a greased baking sheet
5. Bake for 20 min, flipping halfway through cooking time

Tips:

- Serve with a side of homemade apple sauce for dipping
- Can be frozen and reheated for a quick meal option

Nutritional Values: Calories: 220, Fat: 10g, Carbs: 15g, Protein: 18g, Sugar: 2g, Sodium: 200 mg, Potassium: 500 mg, Cholesterol: 80 mg

CUCUMBER SUBMARINE SANDWICHES

Preparation Time: 10 min
Cooking Time: none
Mode of Cooking: No Cooking
Servings: 4
Ingredients:

- 1 large cucumber, cut into 4 equal parts lengthwise, seeds removed
- 8 oz. canned tuna in water, drained
- 1 Tbsp olive oil
- 1 Tbsp lemon juice
- 1/4 red onion, finely chopped
- Salt and pepper to taste
- Fresh dill, chopped

Directions:

1. Hollow out each cucumber piece to create a 'boat'
2. In a bowl, mix tuna, olive oil, lemon juice, chopped red onion, salt, pepper, and dill
3. Spoon tuna mixture into each cucumber boat

Tips:

- Pack with a container of mixed nuts for a satisfying crunch

- Ideal for a low-carb, refreshing lunch option

Nutritional Values: Calories: 180, Fat: 8g, Carbs: 6g, Protein: 20g, Sugar: 3g, Sodium: 210 mg, Potassium: 300 mg, Cholesterol: 30 mg

FRUITY QUINOA SALAD JARS

Preparation Time: 20 min
Cooking Time: 15 min
Mode of Cooking: Boiling
Servings: 4
Ingredients:

- 1 cup quinoa, rinsed and drained
- 2 cups water
- 1 apple, diced
- 1 orange, peeled and segments
- 1/4 cup dried cranberries
- 1/4 cup chopped walnuts
- 3 Tbsp honey
- 2 Tbsp lemon juice
- 1/4 tsp cinnamon

Directions:

1. Rinse quinoa under cold water until water runs clear
2. Bring water to a boil in a saucepan, add quinoa and simmer covered for 15 min until water is absorbed
3. Let quinoa cool
4. In a large bowl, combine cooled quinoa, diced apple, orange segments, cranberries, walnuts, honey, lemon juice, and cinnamon
5. Mix thoroughly

Tips:

- Pack in mason jars for easy transport
- Can be made ahead and stored in the fridge for up to 3 days

Nutritional Values: Calories: 295, Fat: 8g, Carbs: 52g, Protein: 6g, Sugar: 20g, Sodium: 10 mg, Potassium: 400 mg, Cholesterol: 0 mg

RAINBOW VEGGIE WRAPS

Preparation Time: 15 min
Cooking Time: none
Mode of Cooking: No Cooking
Servings: 4
Ingredients:

- 4 large collard green leaves, blanched
- 1 carrot, julienned
- 1 bell pepper, thinly sliced
- 1 small beet, julienned
- 1/2 cucumber, thinly sliced
- 1 avocado, sliced
- 2 Tbsp tahini
- 1 Tbsp lemon juice
- 1/4 tsp garlic powder
- Salt and pepper to taste

Directions:

1. Lay out blanched collard leaves on a flat surface
2. Spread tahini over each leaf
3. Top with carrot, bell pepper, beet, cucumber, and avocado slices evenly distributed
4. Sprinkle with lemon juice, garlic powder, salt, and pepper
5. Roll up tightly and slice into bite-sized pieces

Tips:

- Offer with a side of homemade fruit salsa for added sweetness and dipping fun
- Pack alongside chilled herbal tea for a refreshing lunchbox drink

Nutritional Values: Calories: 250, Fat: 15g, Carbs: 27g, Protein: 8g, Sugar: 5g, Sodium: 150 mg, Potassium: 450 mg, Cholesterol: 0 mg

LEMON HERB MEDITERRANEAN CHICKEN SALAD

Preparation Time: 15 min

Cooking Time: 10 min

Mode of Cooking: Grilling

Servings: 4

Ingredients:

- 2 large boneless skinless chicken breasts
- 2 Tbsp olive oil
- 1 Tbsp lemon zest
- 2 Tbsp lemon juice
- 3 garlic cloves, minced
- 1 tsp dried oregano
- 1 tsp dried thyme
- 1 tsp dried rosemary
- Salt and pepper to taste
- 4 cups mixed greens (such as arugula and spinach)
- 1/2 red onion, thinly sliced
- 1/2 cup cherry tomatoes, halved
- 1/4 cup kalamata olives, pitted
- 1/4 cup cucumber, sliced
- 2 Tbsp capers

Directions:

1. Marinate chicken breasts with olive oil, lemon zest, lemon juice, garlic, oregano, thyme, rosemary, salt, and pepper for 30 min in the refrigerator
2. Heat grill to medium-high heat and grill chicken for 5 min on each side or until fully cooked and juicy
3. Let chicken rest for 5 min then slice
4. Toss mixed greens, onion, tomatoes, olives, cucumber, and capers in a large bowl
5. Top salad with sliced chicken and drizzle with additional olive oil and lemon juice if desired

Tips:

- Serve with a side of grilled whole grain pita for extra fiber
- Add avocado slices for healthy fats and creamy texture

Nutritional Values: Calories: 320, Fat: 14g, Carbs: 12g, Protein: 35g, Sugar: 3g, Sodium: 340 mg, Potassium: 890 mg, Cholesterol: 85 mg

SPICY SHRIMP AND CAULIFLOWER GRITS

Preparation Time: 20 min

Cooking Time: 25 min

Mode of Cooking: Simmering

Servings: 4

Ingredients:

- 1 lb large shrimp, peeled and deveined
- 1 Tbsp paprika
- 1 tsp cayenne pepper
- Salt and pepper to taste
- 2 Tbsp olive oil
- 1 head cauliflower, grated
- 2 cups vegetable broth
- 2 garlic cloves, minced
- 1/2 cup coconut milk
- 1 Tbsp chives, chopped

Directions:

1. Season shrimp with paprika, cayenne, salt, and pepper
2. Heat 1 Tbsp oil in a pan over medium heat and cook shrimp until pink and opaque, about 3-4 min per side, then remove and set aside
3. In the same pan, add remaining oil and sauté garlic until fragrant
4. Add grated cauliflower and vegetable broth, simmer for about 10 min until tender
5. Stir in coconut milk and heat through
6. Serve cauliflower grits topped with spicy shrimp and garnish with chives

Tips:

- Blend additional herbs such as parsley or cilantro into the grits for a fresh flavor boost

• For a less spicy option, reduce cayenne pepper

Nutritional Values: Calories: 295, Fat: 15g, Carbs: 13g, Protein: 25g, Sugar: 5g, Sodium: 300 mg, Potassium: 670 mg, Cholesterol: 180 mg

GARLIC HERB ROASTED SALMON AND VEGGIES

Preparation Time: 10 min
Cooking Time: 20 min
Mode of Cooking: Roasting
Servings: 4
Ingredients:

• 4 salmon fillets
• 2 Tbsp olive oil
• 3 garlic cloves, minced
• 1 Tbsp chopped fresh rosemary
• 1 Tbsp chopped fresh thyme
• Salt and pepper to taste
• 2 cups Brussels sprouts, halved
• 1 cup carrots, sliced
• 1 bell pepper, chopped

Directions:

1. Preheat oven to 425°F (220°C)
2. Mix olive oil with garlic, rosemary, thyme, salt, and pepper
3. Place salmon and vegetables on a baking sheet and drizzle with the herb oil mixture
4. Roast in the oven until salmon is flaky and vegetables are tender, about 20 min

Tips:

• Add a sprinkle of lemon zest over the salmon before serving for a citrusy zing
• Pair with a simple mixed greens salad for extra freshness

Nutritional Values: Calories: 360, Fat: 22g, Carbs: 12g, Protein: 32g, Sugar: 4g, Sodium: 200 mg, Potassium: 950 mg, Cholesterol: 70 mg

TURMERIC CHICKEN AND ROASTED VEGETABLES

Preparation Time: 15 min
Cooking Time: 30 min
Mode of Cooking: Roasting
Servings: 4
Ingredients:

• 4 boneless skinless chicken thighs
• 1 Tbsp turmeric
• 2 Tbsp olive oil
• 1 tsp cumin
• Salt and pepper to taste
• 1/2 head broccoli, chopped
• 2 sweet potatoes, peeled and cubed
• 1 red onion, chopped
• 1 tsp chili flakes

Directions:

1. Preheat oven to 400°F (200°C)
2. Season chicken with turmeric, cumin, salt, pepper, and chili flakes
3. Toss vegetables with olive oil and spread on a baking sheet
4. Place seasoned chicken on top of the vegetables
5. Roast until chicken is golden and cooked through and vegetables are caramelized, about 30 min

Tips:

• Sprinkle with fresh cilantro before serving for a burst of flavor
• Serve with a dollop of Greek yogurt on the side to soften the spice if desired

Nutritional Values: Calories: 410, Fat: 22g, Carbs: 29g, Protein: 27g, Sugar: 7g, Sodium: 310 mg, Potassium: 850 mg, Cholesterol: 110 mg

STUFFED ACORN SQUASH WITH SPICED GROUND TURKEY

Preparation Time: 20 min

Cooking Time: 45 min

Mode of Cooking: Baking

Servings: 4

Ingredients:

- 2 medium acorn squash, halved and seeded
- 1 lb ground turkey
- 1 large onion, finely chopped
- 2 cloves garlic, minced
- 1 tsp ground cinnamon
- 1 tsp smoked paprika
- ½ tsp ground nutmeg
- 2 Tbsp olive oil
- Salt and pepper to taste
- Fresh parsley for garnish

Directions:

1. Preheat oven to 375°F (190°C)
2. Place acorn squash halves cut-side down on a baking sheet and roast for 25 min
3. While squash roasts, heat olive oil in a skillet over medium heat
4. Add onion and garlic, sauté until translucent
5. Add ground turkey, cinnamon, smoked paprika, nutmeg, salt, and pepper, cook until turkey is browned
6. Remove squash from oven, turn cut-side up, and fill with the turkey mixture
7. Return to oven and bake for an additional 20 min
8. Garnish with fresh parsley before serving

Tips:

- Serve with a side of steamed green beans for a complete meal
- Try using ground chicken for a lighter version

Nutritional Values: Calories: 310, Fat: 14g, Carbs: 30g, Protein: 22g, Sugar: 5g, Sodium: 70 mg, Potassium: 980 mg, Cholesterol: 80 mg

CHAPTER 10: SPECIAL OCCASION MEALS

Life is a tapestry of moments, stitched together with memories that sparkle especially brightly when marked by special occasions. Whether you're gathering to celebrate a holiday, host a sophisticated dinner party, or honor a personal milestone like a birthday or an anniversary, food plays a pivotal role in elevating these celebrations into unforgettable experiences.

In this chapter, we delve into the world of special occasion meals, where the essence of whole food cooking merges with the art of festivity. Imagine setting a table that not only looks inviting but is laden with dishes that are as nutritious as they are delectable. It's about striking a balance between tradition and health, without compromising the joy of feasting. So often, we equate special events with indulgence, thinking we need to choose between flavor and well-being. However, with the right recipes and a touch of creativity, you can craft a menu that satisfies both the palate and the body.

From holiday feasts that bring families together around the dining table to elegant entrées that impress the most discerning of guests, the recipes in this chapter are designed to make every occasion both special and healthful. Imagine the delight of your guests as they enjoy a festive feast complete with all the trimmings, knowing that what they're eating is nurturing them as much as it pleases their taste buds.

We'll explore how to prepare sophisticated dishes that harness the rich flavors and abundant nutrients of whole foods, ensuring that even the most lavish meal remains aligned with your health goals. Whether you're planning a large gathering or an intimate soirée, these meals will encourage not only celebration but also a celebration of health.

Let's transform every special occasion into an opportunity for nourishing, jubilant eating that foregrounds wellness without skimping on festivity. After all, every celebration is a chance to feed the soul, foster connections, and create joyous memories, all while sustaining our commitment to a wholesome, vibrant life.

• 10.1 FESTIVE FEASTS

ROSEMARY CITRUS ROAST CHICKEN

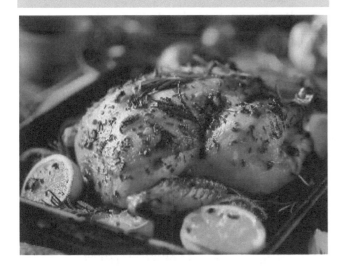

Preparation Time: 15 min.
Cooking Time: 1 hr 30 min.
Mode of Cooking: Roasting

Servings: 4

Ingredients:

- 1 whole chicken (about 4 lb.), rinsed and patted dry
- 1 Tbsp kosher salt
- 2 Tbsp fresh rosemary, chopped
- 4 cloves garlic, minced
- 2 Tbsp ghee, melted
- 1 orange, quartered
- 1 lemon, quartered
- 2 Tbsp olive oil
- Fresh ground black pepper to taste

Directions:

1. Preheat oven to 375°F (190°C)

2. Mix salt, rosemary, garlic, and pepper in a bowl
3. Rub the chicken inside and out with the herb mixture
4. Stuff the cavity with orange and lemon quarters
5. Place chicken in a roasting pan and drizzle with melted ghee and olive oil
6. Roast in the oven until the chicken is golden and juices run clear, about 1 hour and 30 minutes
7. Let rest 10 min. before carving

Tips:

• Carve directly on serving platter to catch all the juices

• Utilize citrus from cavity to squeeze over carved meat for enhanced flavor

Nutritional Values: Calories: 520, Fat: 35g, Carbs: 1g, Protein: 48g, Sugar: 0g, Sodium: 720 mg, Potassium: 360 mg, Cholesterol: 130 mg

SPICED CAULIFLOWER STEAKS WITH WALNUT SAUCE

Preparation Time: 10 min.

Cooking Time: 20 min.

Mode of Cooking: Roasting

Servings: 4

Ingredients:

• 1 large head of cauliflower, sliced into 4 inch thick steaks

• 2 Tbsp olive oil

• 1 tsp turmeric

• 1 tsp ground cumin

• Salt and pepper to taste

• 1 C. walnuts

• 1 clove garlic

• Juice of 1 lemon

• ¼ C. water

• Fresh parsley, chopped for garnish

Directions:

1. Preheat oven to 400°F (200°C)

2. Mix turmeric, cumin, salt, and pepper with olive oil
3. Brush mixture evenly on both sides of cauliflower steaks
4. Roast on a lined baking sheet until tender and golden, about 20 min
5. Blend walnuts, garlic, lemon juice, and water until smooth for sauce
6. Serve steaks drizzled with walnut sauce and garnished with parsley

Tips:

• Serve additional sauce on the side for dipping

• Pair with a crisp white wine to complement the nutty flavors of the dish

Nutritional Values: Calories: 270, Fat: 21g, Carbs: 15g, Protein: 7g, Sugar: 5g, Sodium: 45 mg, Potassium: 860 mg, Cholesterol: 0 mg

HERB-INFUSED WHOLE30 RATATOUILLE

Preparation Time: 20 min.

Cooking Time: 40 min.

Mode of Cooking: Simmering

Servings: 6

Ingredients:

• 2 zucchinis, sliced

• 2 yellow squashes, sliced

• 1 eggplant, cubed

• 3 Roma tomatoes, sliced

• 1 bell pepper, sliced

• 1 onion, sliced

• 3 cloves garlic, minced

• 2 Tbsp olive oil

• 1 tsp dried basil

• 1 tsp dried thyme

• Salt and pepper to taste

• Fresh basil, for garnish

Directions:

1. Preheat your oven to 375°F (190°C)
2. Sauté onions and garlic in olive oil until translucent

3. Add bell pepper and eggplant and cook until beginning to soften
4. Layer the cooked vegetables, zucchini, squash, and tomatoes in a baking dish
5. Season with dried basil, thyme, salt, and pepper
6. Cover and bake for 40 minutes
7. Garnish with fresh basil before serving

Tips:

● Can be made ahead and reheated

● Serve with grilled chicken or fish for a complete meal

● Use a variety of colored vegetables for a vibrant presentation

Nutritional Values: Calories: 115, Fat: 7g, Carbs: 12g, Protein: 2g, Sugar: 7g, Sodium: 10 mg, Potassium: 487 mg, Cholesterol: 0 mg

POMEGRANATE GLAZED LAMB CHOPS

Preparation Time: 15 min.
Cooking Time: 15 min.
Mode of Cooking: Grilling
Servings: 4
Ingredients:

● 8 lamb chops
● Salt and pepper to taste
● 2 Tbsp olive oil
● 1 C. pomegranate juice
● 2 Tbsp balsamic vinegar
● 1 Tbsp honey
● 1 clove garlic, minced
● 1 sprig fresh rosemary
●

Directions:

1. Season lamb chops with salt and pepper
2. Heat olive oil in a skillet and sear lamb chops on high heat for 2-3 min. per side until browned
3. Remove and keep warm
4. In the same skillet, add pomegranate juice, balsamic vinegar, honey, garlic, and rosemary

5. Simmer until reduced by half & thickened into a glaze
6. Brush glaze on lamb chops during last few min. of grilling or roasting
7. Serve hot

Tips:

● Glaze can also be used with beef or grilled chicken

● Fresh pomegranate seeds can be sprinkled on top before serving for added freshness and crunch

Nutritional Values: Calories: 450, Fat: 30g, Carbs: 10g, Protein: 35g, Sugar: 8g, Sodium: 65 mg, Potassium: 515 mg, Cholesterol: 105 mg

POMEGRANATE-GLAZED SALMON WITH DILL

Preparation Time: 20 min
Cooking Time: 15 min
Mode of Cooking: Baking
Servings: 4
Ingredients:

● 4 salmon fillets, each 6 oz.
● 1 cup pomegranate juice
● 2 Tbsp freshly squeezed orange juice
● 1 Tbsp freshly grated ginger
● 2 cloves garlic, minced
● 2 Tbsp fresh dill, chopped
● Sea salt and freshly ground black pepper to taste
● 1 tsp olive oil

Directions:

1. Preheat oven to 375°F (190°C)
2. In a small saucepan, reduce pomegranate juice over medium heat to about 1/3 cup, stir in orange juice, ginger, and garlic, simmer until thickened
3. Brush a baking sheet with olive oil, place salmon fillets, season with salt and pepper, and brush with the pomegranate glaze
4. Bake for 15 min or until salmon flakes easily with a fork
5. Garnish with fresh dill before serving

Tips:

- Serve with a side of steamed asparagus for a complete meal

- Pair with a glass of chilled white wine, such as a Sauvignon Blanc, for an enhanced dining experience

Nutritional Values: Calories: 295, Fat: 13g, Carbs: 11g, Protein: 34g, Sugar: 9g, Sodium: 75 mg, Potassium: 830 mg, Cholesterol: 85 mg

---

• 10.2 ELEGANT ENTREES

STUFFED LAMB WITH SPINACH AND PINE NUTS

Preparation Time: 30 min

Cooking Time: 1 hr

Mode of Cooking: Roasting

Servings: 6

Ingredients:

- 2 lb. lamb shoulder, boned and butterfly-cut
- 1 cup fresh spinach, finely chopped
- ½ cup pine nuts, toasted
- 3 cloves garlic, minced
- 2 Tbsp fresh rosemary, chopped
- 1 Tbsp olive oil
- Salt and pepper to taste
- 1 Tbsp ghee for searing

Directions:

1. Preheat oven to 375°F (190°C)
2. In a bowl, mix spinach, pine nuts, garlic, rosemary, olive oil, salt, and pepper
3. Lay lamb flat and spread filling evenly over the surface
4. Roll lamb tightly and secure with kitchen twine
5. Heat ghee in a pan and sear lamb on all sides until golden
6. Transfer to a roasting pan and roast in the oven for about 1 hr or until desired doneness
7. Let rest for 10 min before slicing

Tips:

- Let the lamb rest before slicing to retain juices

- Serve with a drizzle of rosemary-infused olive oil for added flavor

Nutritional Values: Calories: 450, Fat: 30g, Carbs: 4g, Protein: 40g, Sugar: 1g, Sodium: 120mg, Potassium: 493mg, Cholesterol: 120mg

CEDAR-PLANK SALMON WITH MANGO SALSA

Preparation Time: 20 min

Cooking Time: 20 min

Mode of Cooking: Grilling

Servings: 4

Ingredients:

- 4 salmon fillets, 6 oz each
- 1 large cedar plank, soaked in water for 1 hr
- 1 ripe mango, diced
- ¼ cup red onion, finely chopped
- 1 jalapeño, seeded and minced
- Juice of 1 lime
- 1 Tbsp cilantro, chopped
- Salt and pepper to taste
- 1 Tbsp olive oil

Directions:

1. Preheat grill to medium-high heat
2. In a bowl, combine mango, red onion, jalapeño, lime juice, cilantro, salt, and pepper to make salsa
3. Brush salmon fillets with olive oil and season with salt and pepper
4. Place salmon on soaked cedar plank
5. Grill for about 20 min or until salmon flakes easily
6. Serve hot with mango salsa on top

Tips:

- Soak cedar plank for at least an hour to avoid burning

- Pair with a light, citrusy white wine to complement the flavors of the salsa

Nutritional Values: Calories: 310, Fat: 14g, Carbs: 12g, Protein: 34g, Sugar: 8g, Sodium: 85mg, Potassium: 860mg, Cholesterol: 90mg

HERBED QUAIL WITH BALSAMIC REDUCTION

Preparation Time: 15 min

Cooking Time: 30 min

Mode of Cooking: Roasting

Servings: 4

Ingredients:

- 4 whole quails, cleaned and plucked
- 2 Tbsp fresh thyme, minced
- 2 Tbsp fresh rosemary, minced
- 4 cloves garlic, minced
- 2 Tbsp olive oil
- Salt and pepper to taste
- 1 cup balsamic vinegar
- 1 tsp honey
- 1 Tbsp ghee

Directions:

1. Preheat oven to 400°F (200°C)
2. Mix thyme, rosemary, garlic, and olive oil in a small bowl
3. Rub this mixture all over the quails, inside and out
4. Heat ghee in an oven-safe skillet over medium-high heat
5. Add quails, sear on all sides until golden brown
6. Add balsamic vinegar and honey to the skillet
7. Roast in the oven for about 20 min
8. Baste frequently with pan juices
9. Serve quails drizzled with pan balsamic reduction

Tips:

- Baste quails with the balsamic reduction during roasting to enhance flavor
- Ideal paired with a robust red wine

Nutritional Values: Calories: 410, Fat: 25g, Carbs: 11g, Protein: 35g, Sugar: 9g, Sodium: 60mg, Potassium: 300mg, Cholesterol: 76mg

ROSEMARY AND GARLIC BEEF TENDERLOIN

Preparation Time: 20 min

Cooking Time: 45 min

Mode of Cooking: Roasting

Servings: 8

Ingredients:

- 2½ lb beef tenderloin
- 3 Tbsp fresh rosemary, minced
- 5 cloves garlic, minced
- 2 Tbsp olive oil
- 2 tsp coarse sea salt
- 1 tsp ground black pepper
- 1 cup red wine

Directions:

1. Preheat oven to 400°F (200°C)
2. Combine rosemary, garlic, olive oil, salt, and pepper in a small bowl
3. Rub mixture liberally all over beef tenderloin
4. Place tenderloin in a roasting pan
5. Roast for 45 min or until meat reaches desired level of doneness
6. Halfway through, pour red wine over the beef
7. Let rest for 15 min before slicing

Tips:

- Pouring wine over beef while cooking adds flavor and keeps it moist
- Rest beef before slicing to ensure juices redistribute
- Pair with a full-bodied red wine to match the robust flavors of the dish

Nutritional Values: Calories: 360, Fat: 22g, Carbs: 1g, Protein: 35g, Sugar: 0g, Sodium: 590mg, Potassium: 500mg, Cholesterol: 90mg

SEARED SCALLOPS WITH CAULIFLOWER PURÉE AND ASPARAGUS

Preparation Time: 15 min.

Cooking Time: 15 min.

Mode of Cooking: Sautéing and Boiling

Servings: 4

Ingredients:

- 12 large sea scallops, cleaned
- 1 head cauliflower, cut into florets

- 1 lb asparagus, trimmed
- 3 Tbsp. extra virgin olive oil
- 1 tsp. garlic powder
- Salt and fresh ground black pepper to taste
- Fresh parsley for garnishing

Directions:

1. Bring a pot of lightly salted water to a boil and add cauliflower florets, cooking until tender, about 10 min.
2. Drain and blend cauliflower in a food processor until smooth, adding 2 Tbsp. olive oil, garlic powder, and season with salt and pepper
3. While cauliflower cooks, heat the remaining oil in a pan over medium-high heat and sear scallops for about 2 min. on each side until a golden crust forms
4. Steam asparagus until tender-crisp, about 3-4 min.
5. To serve, spread cauliflower purée on plates, top with scallops and arrange asparagus

Tips:

- Garnish with fresh parsley for a touch of color and freshness
- Ensure scallops are dry before searing to get a good crust
- Do not overcrowd the scallops in the pan to allow proper searing

Nutritional Values: Calories: 240, Fat: 10g, Carbs: 14g, Protein: 23g, Sugar: 3g, Sodium: 320 mg, Potassium: 620 mg, Cholesterol: 40 mg

• 10.3 FUN AND FESTIVE

SPICED CITRUS & HERB GRILLED CHICKEN SKEWERS

Preparation Time: 20 min
Cooking Time: 15 min
Mode of Cooking: Grilling
Servings: 4

Ingredients:

- 2 lbs chicken breast, cut into 1-inch cubes
- 3 Tbsp extra virgin olive oil
- 2 cloves garlic, minced
- 1 orange, zested and juiced
- 1 lemon, zested and juiced
- 1 Tbsp fresh rosemary, minced
- 1 Tbsp fresh thyme, minced
- 1 tsp smoked paprika
- 1 tsp sea salt
- 1/2 tsp black pepper

Directions:

1. Combine olive oil, garlic, orange zest, orange juice, lemon zest, lemon juice, rosemary, thyme, smoked paprika, salt, and pepper in a bowl
2. Add chicken cubes to the marinade and let sit for at least 15 minutes
3. Thread chicken onto skewers
4. Grill over medium heat, turning occasionally, until chicken is cooked thoroughly and has nice grill marks, about 15 min

Tips:

- Marinate overnight for deeper flavor
- Serve with a side of grilled vegetables
- Use metal skewer for best results

Nutritional Values: Calories: 310, Fat: 13g, Carbs: 6g, Protein: 40g, Sugar: 2g, Sodium: 620 mg, Potassium: 300 mg, Cholesterol: 98 mg

ROASTED CAULIFLOWER AND POMEGRANATE SALAD

Preparation Time: 15 min
Cooking Time: 25 min
Mode of Cooking: Roasting
Servings: 6
Ingredients:

- 1 large head cauliflower, cut into bite-sized florets
- 1 Tbsp coconut oil, melted
- 1 tsp cumin

- 1/2 tsp sea salt
- 1/4 tsp black pepper
- 1 pomegranate, seeded
- 1/4 C. fresh parsley, chopped
- 3 Tbsp extra virgin olive oil
- 2 Tbsp lemon juice

Directions:

1. Toss cauliflower florets with melted coconut oil, cumin, salt, and pepper, and spread on a baking sheet
2. Roast in preheated oven at 425°F (220°C) until golden and tender, about 25 min
3. In a large bowl, combine roasted cauliflower, pomegranate seeds, and chopped parsley
4. Drizzle with olive oil and lemon juice, and toss to combine

Tips:

- Serve warm or at room temperature
- Add crumbled feta if not on Whole30
- Can be prepared ahead and stored in the refrigerator

Nutritional Values: Calories: 150, Fat: 10g, Carbs: 15g, Protein: 3g, Sugar: 9g, Sodium: 200 mg, Potassium: 470 mg, Cholesterol: 0 mg

FESTIVE STUFFED BELL PEPPERS

Preparation Time: 30 min
Cooking Time: 45 min
Mode of Cooking: Baking
Servings: 4
Ingredients:

- 4 large bell peppers, assorted colors, tops cut off and seeded
- 1 lb turkey mince
- 1/2 C. diced onions
- 2 cloves garlic, minced
- 1 tsp cumin
- 1 tsp chili powder
- 1/2 tsp sea salt
- 1/4 tsp black pepper
- 1 C. diced tomatoes
- 1/4 C. fresh cilantro, chopped
- Coconut oil for greasing

Directions:

1. Sauté onions and garlic in a skillet with a bit of coconut oil until translucent
2. Add turkey mince, breaking it up with a spoon till browned
3. Stir in cumin, chili powder, salt, and pepper and cook for another 2 min
4. Remove from heat and add diced tomatoes and cilantro
5. Fill each pepper with the turkey mixture
6. Place in a pre-greased baking dish and bake at 375°F (190°C) for 45 min

Tips:

- These can be made ahead and reheated
- Top with avocado slices or a scoop of salsa for extra freshness
- Great for a make-ahead meal prep

Nutritional Values: Calories: 260, Fat: 12g, Carbs: 18g, Protein: 22g, Sugar: 8g, Sodium: 580 mg, Potassium: 650 mg, Cholesterol: 80 mg

AVOCADO & MANGO SALSA

Preparation Time: 10 min
Cooking Time: none
Mode of Cooking: Mixing
Servings: 5
Ingredients:

- 2 ripe avocados, diced
- 1 ripe mango, diced
- 1/4 C. red onion, finely chopped
- 1 small jalapeño, seeds removed and finely diced
- 1/4 C. fresh cilantro, chopped
- Juice of 1 lime
- 1/2 tsp sea salt
- 1/4 tsp black pepper

Directions:

1. Combine all ingredients in a bowl and gently mix to combine without smashing the avocado

2. Serve immediately or chill in the refrigerator to let flavors meld for about an hour

Tips:

- Perfect as a dip or to top off any grilled meat
- Adding a bit of diced cucumber can provide a refreshing crunch
- Keep the seed of the avocado in the bowl to prevent browning

Nutritional Values: Calories: 140, Fat: 9g, Carbs: 15g, Protein: 2g, Sugar: 5g, Sodium: 240 mg, Potassium: 360 mg, Cholesterol: 0 mg

RAINBOW VEGGIE KABOBS WITH AVOCADO DIPPING SAUCE

Preparation Time: 15 min

Cooking Time: 10 min

Mode of Cooking: Grilling

Servings: 4

Ingredients:

- 3 medium zucchinis, sliced into ½ inch rounds
- 2 large red bell peppers, cut into 1 inch pieces
- 2 large yellow bell peppers, cut into 1 inch pieces
- 2 large orange bell peppers, cut into 1 inch pieces
- 1 large red onion, cut into wedges
- 1 pint cherry tomatoes
- 2 Tbsp extra virgin olive oil
- 1 tsp garlic powder
- 1 tsp onion powder
- Salt and pepper to taste
- For the sauce: 1 ripe avocado
- 1 clove garlic, minced
- Juice of 1 lime
- ¼ cup coconut cream
- Salt and pepper to taste

Directions:

1. Thread the vegetables alternately onto skewers
2. Brush with olive oil and season with garlic powder, onion powder, salt, and pepper
3. Grill over medium heat, turning occasionally, until vegetables are tender and slightly charred, about 10 min
4. For the sauce: Blend avocado, garlic, lime juice, coconut cream, salt, and pepper until smooth

Tips:

- Serve kabobs immediately with avocado dipping sauce for a fresh, festive touch
- If not using wooden skewers, pre-soak them in water for 30 min to avoid burning on the grill
- The dipping sauce can be refrigerated for up to 2 days

Nutritional Values: Calories: 180, Fat: 12g, Carbs: 18g, Protein: 4g, Sugar: 9g, Sodium: 60mg, Potassium: 560mg, Cholesterol: 0mg

CHAPTER 11: EATING ON A BUDGET

Imagine this: You're wading through the supermarket aisles, your grocery list in one hand and a calculator in the other, meticulously adding up prices and occasionally sighing at the cost of health-conscious options. It's a common scene for many who strive to feed their families nutritious meals on a tight budget. The good news? Eating wholesome, whole food meals doesn't have to be a luxury reserved for those with flexible budgets.

In this chapter, we'll dispel the myth that healthy eating is prohibitively expensive. With a little knowledge and some creative planning, you can enjoy delicious, nutrient-packed meals without stretching your wallet too thin. Think of it as your guide to being an economical gourmet, combining the art of healthy eating with the science of budget management.

First, let's address a crucial mindset shift: viewing budgeting as an opportunity rather than a constraint. Each dollar saved is a step towards financial freedom, and every nutritious meal prepared cost-effectively is a victory for your health. It's all about making smart choices—selecting ingredients that offer the best nutritional bang for your buck, utilizing local and seasonal produce, and mastering the art of meal planning and prep.

We'll explore techniques to minimize food waste, which will not only save money but also contribute to environmental sustainability. You'll learn how to transform leftovers into new culinary creations, and how to use every part of an ingredient for maximum benefit.

By the end of this chapter, the vision of navigating those supermarket aisles with confidence and creativity, stretching each dollar while enriching your diet with quality whole foods, will seem not just possible, but exciting. The journey to a healthier lifestyle, irrespective of your budget constraints, begins with this new perspective. Let's embark on this journey together, turning economic limitations into a canvas for culinary innovation.

• 11.1 BUDGET BREAKFASTS

SPICED PUMPKIN BREAKFAST PORRIDGE

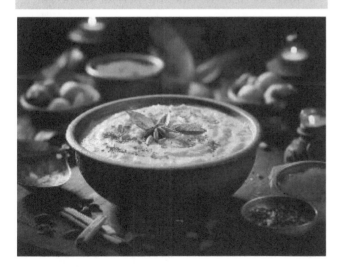

Preparation Time: 5 min
Cooking Time: 15 min
Mode of Cooking: Stovetop
Servings: 2

Ingredients:

- 1 cup canned pumpkin puree
- 1 ½ cups coconut milk
- 1 tsp ground cinnamon
- ½ tsp ground nutmeg
- ¼ tsp ground ginger
- 1 Tbsp chia seeds
- 1 Tbsp flaxseed meal
- Pinch of salt
- Optional toppings: sliced almonds, coconut flakes

Directions:

1. Combine pumpkin puree, coconut milk, cinnamon, nutmeg, ginger, and salt in a saucepan over medium heat
2. Stir in chia seeds and flaxseed meal

3. Cook, stirring occasionally, until the mixture thickens and is heated through, about 15 min
4. Serve hot with optional toppings of sliced almonds and coconut flakes

Tips:

- Use light coconut milk for a lower fat version
- Top with seasonal fruits for added freshness and flavor

Nutritional Values: Calories: 287, Fat: 17g, Carbs: 27g, Protein: 5g, Sugar: 12g, Sodium: 30 mg, Potassium: 264 mg, Cholesterol: 0 mg

SAVORY MUSHROOM AND SPINACH FRITTATA

Preparation Time: 10 min
Cooking Time: 20 min
Mode of Cooking: Oven
Servings: 4
Ingredients:

- 4 eggs
- 1 cup fresh spinach, chopped
- ½ cup mushrooms, sliced
- 2 Tbsp ghee
- ¼ tsp salt
- ¼ tsp black pepper
- ¼ cup water

Directions:

1. Preheat oven to 375°F (190°C)
2. In a skillet, heat ghee over medium heat and sauté mushrooms until soft
3. Add spinach and cook until wilted
4. In a bowl, whisk together eggs, water, salt, and pepper
5. Pour egg mixture over the vegetables in the skillet
6. Transfer skillet to preheated oven and bake until eggs are set, about 20 min

Tips:

- Serve with a side of avocado for healthy fats
- Can be stored in the refrigerator and reheated for a quick breakfast

Nutritional Values: Calories: 160, Fat: 12g, Carbs: 3g, Protein: 9g, Sugar: 1g, Sodium: 300 mg, Potassium: 230 mg, Cholesterol: 215 mg

ZESTY AVOCADO AND TOMATO SALAD

Preparation Time: 10 min
Cooking Time: none
Mode of Cooking: No Cooking
Servings: 2
Ingredients:

- 1 large ripe avocado, cubed
- 1 cup cherry tomatoes, halved
- ¼ cup red onion, finely chopped
- 1 Tbsp olive oil
- 1 Tbsp lime juice
- Salt and pepper to taste

Directions:

1. In a mixing bowl, combine all ingredients
2. Gently toss to coat the avocado and tomatoes with olive oil and lime juice

Tips:

- Season with salt and pepper to enhance flavors just before serving
- Rich in healthy fats and perfect for a quick, energizing start

Nutritional Values: Calories: 250, Fat: 21g, Carbs: 17g, Protein: 3g, Sugar: 3g, Sodium: 10 mg, Potassium: 690 mg, Cholesterol: 0 mg

SUNRISE SWEET POTATO HASH

Preparation Time: 10 min.
Cooking Time: 15 min.
Mode of Cooking: Sauteeing
Servings: 4
Ingredients:

- 1 large sweet potato, peeled and diced
- 1 red bell pepper, diced
- 1 medium onion, diced
- 2 cloves garlic, minced
- 4 eggs

- 1 Tbsp olive oil
- salt and pepper to taste
- 1/4 tsp smoked paprika

Directions:

1. Heat olive oil in a large skillet over medium heat
2. Add sweet potato, bell pepper, and onion and cook until tender, about 10 minutes
3. Make four wells in the hash, crack an egg into each well, cover the skillet, and cook until eggs are set, about 5 minutes
4. Season with salt, pepper, and smoked paprika

Tips:

- Serve with a sprinkle of fresh herbs such as parsley for enhanced flavor
- This recipe can be easily doubled for meal prep or larger families
- For extra protein, add chopped cooked chicken or turkey

Nutritional Values: Calories: 210, Fat: 10g, Carbs: 23g, Protein: 9g, Sugar: 5g, Sodium: 125 mg, Potassium: 330 mg, Cholesterol: 165 mg

BANANA NUT OATMEAL

Preparation Time: 5 min.

Cooking Time: 10 min.

Mode of Cooking: Boiling

Servings: 2

Ingredients:

- 1 C. rolled oats
- 1 banana, sliced
- 2 Tbsp walnuts, chopped
- 1 Tbsp flaxseeds
- 1/2 tsp cinnamon
- 2 C. water
- pinch of salt

Directions:

1. Bring water to a boil in a small saucepan
2. Add oats and salt, reduce heat, and simmer for 5 minutes, stirring occasionally

3. Remove from heat, stir in sliced banana, chopped walnuts, flaxseeds, and cinnamon

Tips:

- Add a spoonful of almond butter for creaminess and extra protein
- Customize with other fruits like berries or peaches for variety and added nutrients

Nutritional Values: Calories: 307, Fat: 11g, Carbs: 45g, Protein: 9g, Sugar: 7g, Sodium: 30 mg, Potassium: 250 mg, Cholesterol: 0 mg

• 11.2 LUNCH ON LESS

ZESTY TUNA AND AVOCADO SALAD

Preparation Time: 15 min

Cooking Time: none

Mode of Cooking: No Cooking

Servings: 4

Ingredients:

- 2 cans tuna in water, drained
- 2 ripe avocados, cubed
- 1 small red onion, finely chopped
- 1 red bell pepper, diced
- 1 cucumber, diced
- Juice of 2 limes
- 1 tsp dried oregano
- Salt and pepper to taste
- 2 Tbsp olive oil

Directions:

1. Combine tuna, avocados, red onion, bell pepper, and cucumber in a large bowl
2. In a small bowl, whisk together lime juice, oregano, salt, pepper, and olive oil
3. Pour dressing over tuna mixture and gently toss to combine

Tips:

- Opt for chunk light tuna in water for a leaner, cost-effective option
- Lime can be substituted with vinegar for a different tangy twist

- Chill before serving to enhance flavors

Nutritional Values: Calories: 290, Fat: 19g, Carbs: 12g, Protein: 22g, Sugar: 2g, Sodium: 210 mg, Potassium: 450 mg, Cholesterol: 30 mg

SPICY CHICKPEA STEW

Preparation Time: 10 min
Cooking Time: 20 min
Mode of Cooking: Stovetop
Servings: 6
Ingredients:

- 1 Tbsp coconut oil
- 1 large onion, chopped
- 3 cloves garlic, minced
- 1 Tbsp ginger, grated
- 1 Tbsp curry powder
- 1 tsp cumin
- 1 tsp paprika
- 1 can chickpeas, drained and rinsed
- 1 can diced tomatoes
- 4 cups vegetable broth
- Salt and pepper to taste
- Fresh cilantro for garnish

Directions:

1. Heat coconut oil in a large pot over medium heat
2. Add onion, garlic, and ginger, sauté until onion is translucent
3. Stir in curry powder, cumin, and paprika and cook for 1 min
4. Add chickpeas, tomatoes, and vegetable broth, bring to a boil, then simmer for 20 min
5. Season with salt and pepper, garnish with cilantro before serving

Tips:

- Serve with a side of baked sweet potatoes for a hearty meal
- Leftovers can be refrigerated and taste even better the next day

Nutritional Values: Calories: 180, Fat: 4g, Carbs: 29g, Protein: 9g, Sugar: 5g, Sodium: 300 mg, Potassium: 470 mg, Cholesterol: 0 mg

SQUASH AND APPLE SOUP

Preparation Time: 15 min
Cooking Time: 25 min
Mode of Cooking: Stovetop
Servings: 4
Ingredients:

- 1 Tbsp olive oil
- 1 butternut squash, peeled and cubed
- 2 apples, peeled and chopped
- 1 onion, chopped
- 4 cups chicken broth
- 1 tsp cinnamon
- Salt and pepper to taste
- Greek yogurt for topping (optional)

Directions:

1. Heat olive oil in a large pot over medium heat
2. Add squash, apples, and onion, cook until slightly soft ♫ Add broth and bring to a boil
3. Reduce heat and simmer until squash is tender, about 20 min
4. Puree with an immersion blender until smooth
5. Stir in cinnamon, salt, and pepper
6. Serve hot, topped with a dollop of Greek yogurt

Tips:

- For a vegan version, substitute chicken broth with vegetable broth and skip the yogurt topping
- Cinnamon can be replaced with nutmeg for a different flavor profile

Nutritional Values: Calories: 150, Fat: 3g, Carbs: 31g, Protein: 3g, Sugar: 14g, Sodium: 480 mg, Potassium: 800 mg, Cholesterol: 0 mg

LEMONY LENTIL AND RICE SALAD

Preparation Time: 20 min

Cooking Time: 30 min

Mode of Cooking: Stovetop

Servings: 6

Ingredients:

- 1 cup brown rice
- 1 cup green lentils
- 1 lemon, zest and juice
- 1 cucumber, diced
- 1 bell pepper, diced
- 1/4 cup chopped fresh parsley
- 1/4 cup olive oil
- Salt and pepper to taste

Directions:

1. Cook rice and lentils separately according to package instructions until tender
2. In a large bowl, combine cooked rice, lentils, lemon zest, and juice, cucumber, bell pepper, and parsley
3. Drizzle with olive oil, season with salt and pepper, and toss well

Tips:

- This salad can be served either warm or cold
- Lemon zest adds a refreshing zestiness, adjust according to taste
- Incorporate diced tomatoes for added freshness and flavor

Nutritional Values: Calories: 220, Fat: 7g, Carbs: 33g, Protein: 9g, Sugar: 3g, Sodium: 10 mg, Potassium: 320 mg, Cholesterol: 0 mg

SPICY TUNA STUFFED AVOCADO

Preparation Time: 10 min.

Cooking Time: none

Mode of Cooking: No Cooking

Servings: 2

Ingredients:

- 1 large avocado, halved and pitted
- 1 can (5 oz.) tuna, drained
- 1/4 red onion, finely chopped
- 1 Tbsp. jalapeño, minced
- 1 Tbsp. cilantro, chopped
- 1 Tbsp. lime juice
- Salt and pepper to taste

Directions:

1. Scoop out some of the avocado from the pits to make room for the filling
2. In a bowl, mix tuna, red onion, jalapeño, cilantro, and lime juice
3. Season the mixture with salt and pepper
4. Spoon the tuna mixture into the avocado halves

Tips:

- Use ripe avocados for the best texture
- Add a dash of chili flakes if you prefer more heat

Nutritional Values: Calories: 300, Fat: 22g, Carbs: 15g, Protein: 13g, Sugar: 2g, Sodium: 70 mg, Potassium: 450 mg, Cholesterol: 30 mg

---

• 11.3 ECONOMICAL DINNERS

RUSTIC CHICKEN & VEGETABLE TRAYBAKE

Preparation Time: 15 min

Cooking Time: 40 min

Mode of Cooking: Baking

Servings: 4

Ingredients:

- 2 lb. bone-in, skin-on chicken thighs
- 1 lb. carrots, peeled and cut into sticks
- 1 lb. parsnips, peeled and cut into sticks
- 1 large onion, sliced
- 4 cloves garlic, minced
- 2 Tbsp olive oil
- 1 tsp dried thyme
- 1 tsp dried rosemary
- Salt and pepper to taste

Directions:

1. Preheat oven to 425°F (220°C)

2. In a large mixing bowl, toss carrots, parsnips, onion, and garlic with olive oil, thyme, rosemary, salt, and pepper
3. Spread the vegetables evenly on a baking tray
4. Place chicken thighs on top of the vegetables
5. Bake in the preheated oven for 40 min or until chicken is golden and veggies are tender

Tips:

- Use parchment paper for easy cleanup
- Leftover veggies can be pureed into a soup
- Experiment with different herbs like sage or oregano for variety

Nutritional Values: Calories: 350, Fat: 22g, Carbs: 15g, Protein: 24g, Sugar: 5g, Sodium: 70 mg, Potassium: 320 mg, Cholesterol: 80 mg

SPICED PORK TENDERLOIN WITH CAULIFLOWER RICE

Preparation Time: 10 min
Cooking Time: 25 min
Mode of Cooking: Roasting
Servings: 4
Ingredients:

- 1 pork tenderloin, about 1 lb
- 2 Tbsp smoked paprika
- 1 tsp garlic powder
- 1 tsp onion powder
- Salt and pepper to taste
- 1 head of cauliflower, chopped
- 2 Tbsp coconut oil
- 1 Tbsp chopped fresh cilantro

Directions:

1. Preheat oven to 375°F (190°C)
2. Rub the pork tenderloin with smoked paprika, garlic powder, onion powder, salt, and pepper
3. Heat coconut oil in a skillet over medium heat and brown the pork on all sides
4. Transfer to a baking sheet and roast for 20 min

5. Meanwhile, sauté the cauliflower rice in the same skillet for 5 min
6. Garnish with fresh cilantro

Tips:

- Let pork rest for 5 min before slicing
- Cauliflower rice can be flavored with lime zest for extra zing
- Serve with a simple side salad for additional freshness

Nutritional Values: Calories: 250, Fat: 15g, Carbs: 8g, Protein: 22g, Sugar: 3g, Sodium: 65 mg, Potassium: 600 mg, Cholesterol: 65 mg

LEMON-HERB BAKED COD WITH ZUCCHINI NOODLES

Preparation Time: 10 min
Cooking Time: 15 min
Mode of Cooking: Baking
Servings: 4
Ingredients:

- 4 cod fillets, about 6 oz each
- 2 lemons, zested and juiced
- 3 Tbsp olive oil
- 1 Tbsp dried dill
- 1 Tbsp dried parsley
- Salt and pepper to taste
- 4 medium zucchini, spiralized into noodles
- 1 Tbsp ghee

Directions:

1. Preheat oven to 400°F (200°C)
2. Mix lemon zest, lemon juice, olive oil, dill, parsley, salt, and pepper together
3. Lay cod fillets on a greased baking dish
4. Pour the lemon-herb mixture over the cod
5. Bake for 15 min
6. Sauté the zucchini noodles in ghee for about 5 min until tender

Tips:

- Serve cod over zucchini noodles
- Add capers to the lemon sauce for extra tang
- Keep the skin on zucchini for added nutrients

Nutritional Values: Calories: 200, Fat: 10g, Carbs: 6g, Protein: 20g, Sugar: 3g, Sodium: 80 mg, Potassium: 500 mg, Cholesterol: 60 mg

RUSTIC CHICKEN AND VEGETABLE BAKE

Preparation Time: 15 min
Cooking Time: 45 min
Mode of Cooking: Baking
Servings: 4
Ingredients:

- 2 lbs. chicken thighs, bone-in and skin on
- 3 medium carrots, sliced
- 2 parsnips, sliced
- 1 large onion, quartered
- 4 cloves garlic, minced
- 3 Tbsp olive oil
- 1 tsp dried thyme
- 1 tsp dried rosemary
- Salt and pepper to taste

Directions:

1. Preheat oven to 375°F (190°C)
2. Toss all vegetables with olive oil, garlic, thyme, rosemary, salt, and pepper in a large baking dish
3. Nestle the chicken thighs among the vegetables
4. Bake in the preheated oven until chicken is golden and vegetables are tender, about 45 min

Tips:

- Use chicken legs for a cheaper alternative
- Incorporate any seasonal vegetables available at a lower cost

Nutritional Values: Calories: 520, Fat: 35g, Carbs: 20g, Protein: 32g, Sugar: 6g, Sodium: 120 mg, Potassium: 650 mg, Cholesterol: 140 mg

SPICY TUNA AND BROCCOLI STIR-FRY

Preparation Time: 10 min
Cooking Time: 15 min
Mode of Cooking: Stir-frying
Servings: 4
Ingredients:

- 2 cans of tuna in water, drained
- 2 heads of broccoli, cut into florets
- 1 red bell pepper, sliced
- 2 Tbsp coconut oil
- 2 Tbsp soy sauce (or coconut aminos)
- 1 tsp chili flakes
- 1 tsp ginger, grated
- Salt to taste

Directions:

1. Heat coconut oil in a large skillet over medium-high heat
2. Add broccoli and bell pepper, stir-fry for about 5 min until they start to soften
3. Add tuna, soy sauce, chili flakes, and ginger
4. Cook for an additional 5-10 min, stirring occasionally until everything is heated through and nicely combined

Tips:

- Opt for frozen broccoli to reduce costs and prep time
- Tuna can be swapped for any leftover cooked meat

Nutritional Values: Calories: 180, Fat: 8g, Carbs: 9g, Protein: 20g, Sugar: 3g, Sodium: 630 mg, Potassium: 450 mg, Cholesterol: 30 mg

CHAPTER 12: WORLD OF FLAVORS

Embark with me on a gustatory journey around the globe, from the sun-drenched coasts of the Mediterranean to the vibrant markets of Asia and the festive spirit of Latin America. In this chapter, we explore the endless flavors and wholesome traditions of world cuisines, each recipe carefully curated not only to excite your taste buds but also to nourish your body with nature's best.

Imagine walking through a bustling market, the air fragrant with spices and fresh herbs, your senses dazzled by the colors of freshly harvested vegetables and fruits. This is the essence of eating whole foods—a celebration of life's natural bounty which transcends geographical boundaries. Our culinary adventure is more than just a tour of global dishes; it's an invitation to weave the rich tapestries of international food culture into your daily meals, making each bite a testament to health and happiness.

Consider the timeless appeal of a Greek salad, the vibrancy of a Thai stir-fry, or the comforting warmth of an Italian minestrone. These dishes do more than satiate hunger—they offer a connection to the world at large, promoting a diet that's as good for the planet as it is for your plate. Each recipe in this chapter promises simplicity and satisfaction, leveraging the power of whole ingredients that pack a nutritional punch, without requiring hours of preparation or hard-to-find components.

As we venture through these pages, I encourage you to embrace the diversity of meals that have brought families together across the globe. Let each meal be an opportunity for exploration and joy, proving that healthy eating doesn't have to be restrictive or mundane—it can be a vibrant celebration of global heritage and personal well-being. Join me in bringing the world to your kitchen, where every dish tells a story and every ingredient plays a starring role in your journey toward better health.

• 12.1 INTERNATIONAL INSPIRATIONS

MOROCCAN HARIRA SOUP

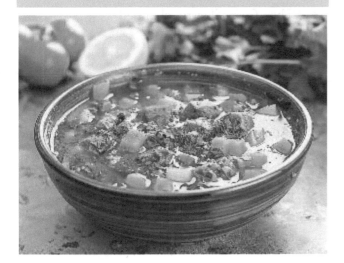

Preparation Time: 20 min.
Cooking Time: 60 min.
Mode of Cooking: Stovetop
Servings: 6

Ingredients:
- 8 oz. lean lamb, cubed
- 3 large tomatoes, peeled and diced
- 1 large onion, diced
- 2 celery stalks, chopped
- 2 carrots, diced
- 1 bunch cilantro, chopped
- 1 bunch parsley, chopped
- 4 cups bone broth
- 1 Tbsp turmeric
- 1 tsp cumin
- 1 tsp cinnamon
- 1 Tbsp olive oil
- 1 tsp black pepper
- 2 cups water
- 1 lemon, juiced

Directions:

1. Heat olive oil in a large pot over medium heat
2. Sauté onions, celery, and carrots until tender
3. Add lamb and brown slightly
4. Mix in tomatoes, spices, and herbs, stirring for 2 min.
5. Pour in bone broth and water, bring to a boil, then reduce to a simmer for 50 min.
6. Just before serving, stir in lemon juice

Tips:

- Serve with a wedge of lemon for added zest
- Top with fresh cilantro for enhanced flavor

Nutritional Values: Calories: 240, Fat: 10g, Carbs: 20g, Protein: 17g, Sugar: 5g, Sodium: 80 mg, Potassium: 700 mg, Cholesterol: 50 mg

THAI BASIL CHICKEN (GAI PAD KRAPOW)

Preparation Time: 15 min.

Cooking Time: 10 min.

Mode of Cooking: Stovetop

Servings: 4

Ingredients:

- 1 lb. ground chicken
- 2 cups Thai basil leaves
- 4 cloves garlic, minced
- 3 bird's eye chilies, minced
- 1 red bell pepper, sliced
- 1 Tbsp fish sauce
- 1 Tbsp coconut aminos
- 2 tsp coconut oil
- 1 Tbsp fresh lime juice
- 1 tsp raw honey (optional, omit for stricter Whole30)

Directions:

1. Heat coconut oil in a skillet over medium-high heat
2. Sauté garlic and chilies until fragrant
3. Add chicken and cook thoroughly
4. Stir in bell pepper, fish sauce, coconut aminos, and lime juice
5. Cook until pepper softens
6. Remove from heat and stir in basil leaves until wilted

Tips:

- Opt for fresh Thai basil for authentic flavor
- Adjust chili quantity based on spice preference

Nutritional Values: Calories: 235, Fat: 13g, Carbs: 8g, Protein: 22g, Sugar: 4g (omit honey), Sodium: 620 mg, Potassium: 415 mg, Cholesterol: 98 mg

INDIAN SPICED ROASTED CAULIFLOWER

Preparation Time: 10 min.

Cooking Time: 25 min.

Mode of Cooking: Oven Roasting

Servings: 4

Ingredients:

- 1 head cauliflower, cut into florets
- 2 Tbsp ghee, melted
- 1 tsp turmeric
- 1 tsp garam masala
- 1 tsp coriander
- ½ tsp cumin
- ½ tsp salt
- ¼ tsp black pepper
- 1 lime, juiced
- 2 Tbsp fresh cilantro, chopped

Directions:

1. Preheat oven to 425°F (220°C)
2. Mix ghee, turmeric, garam masala, coriander, cumin, salt, and pepper in a large bowl
3. Add cauliflower florets and toss to coat evenly
4. Spread on a baking sheet and roast for 25 min.
5. Sprinkle lime juice and cilantro before serving

Tips:

- Use parchment paper for easy cleanup
- Serve alongside a protein like grilled chicken for a complete meal

Nutritional Values: Calories: 120, Fat: 9g, Carbs: 10g, Protein: 3g, Sugar: 4g, Sodium: 300 mg, Potassium: 470 mg, Cholesterol: 20 mg

BRAZILIAN MOQUECA (FISH STEW)

Preparation Time: 20 min.

Cooking Time: 40 min.

Mode of Cooking: Stovetop

Servings: 6

Ingredients:

- 1.5 lbs. firm white fish, such as cod, cubed
- 1 large onion, sliced
- 1 red bell pepper, sliced
- 1 yellow bell pepper, sliced
- 3 cloves garlic, minced
- 2 Tbsp lime juice
- 2 cups coconut milk
- 2 tbsp olive oil
- 1 tsp paprika
- 1 Tbsp fresh cilantro, chopped
- 2 tomatoes, diced
- 1 chili pepper, sliced
- Salt to taste
- Black pepper to taste

Directions:

1. Heat olive oil in a large pot over medium heat
2. Sauté onion, bell peppers, and garlic until soft
3. Add tomatoes, chili pepper, and paprika, cook for 5 min.
4. Pour in coconut milk and bring to a simmer
5. Add the fish and simmer gently for 25 min.
6. Finish with lime juice and cilantro before serving

Tips:

- Serve with cauliflower rice for a complete Whole30 meal
- Adjust the heat level by increasing or decreasing the amount of chili pepper

Nutritional Values: Calories: 350, Fat: 22g, Carbs: 12g, Protein: 28g, Sugar: 5g, Sodium: 85 mg, Potassium: 860 mg, Cholesterol: 65 mg

THAI COCONUT CHICKEN SOUP

Preparation Time: 15 min

Cooking Time: 30 min

Mode of Cooking: Stovetop

Servings: 4

Ingredients:

- 1 Tbsp coconut oil
- 1 lb chicken breast, thinly sliced
- 1 large onion, sliced
- 2 cloves garlic, minced
- 1 Tbsp fresh ginger, grated
- 2 Tbsp Thai red curry paste
- 4 cups chicken broth
- 1 can (14 oz) coconut milk
- 1 Tbsp fish sauce
- 2 tsp lime juice
- 1 cup shiitake mushrooms, sliced
- 1 red bell pepper, julienned
- 1/2 cup fresh cilantro, chopped
- Salt to taste

Directions:

1. Heat coconut oil in a large pot over medium heat
2. Add chicken and onion, sauté until chicken is browned and onions are soft
3. Add garlic, ginger, and red curry paste, cook for 2 minutes
4. Pour in chicken broth, bring to a boil
5. Add coconut milk, fish sauce, and lime juice, reduce heat to simmer for 20 minutes
6. Add mushrooms and red pepper, cook for an additional 10 minutes
7. Garnish with fresh cilantro and season with salt

Tips:

- Use homemade chicken broth for richer flavor
- Add a dash of chili oil for extra spice

Nutritional Values: Calories: 310, Fat: 18g, Carbs: 9g, Protein: 28g, Sugar: 4g, Sodium: 750 mg, Potassium: 800 mg, Cholesterol: 90 mg

Greek Style Cauliflower Salad

Preparation Time: 15 min

Cooking Time: none

Mode of Cooking: No Cooking

Servings: 4

Ingredients:

- 1 head cauliflower, chopped
- 1 cup cherry tomatoes, halved
- 1 cucumber, diced
- 1/2 cup red onion, thinly sliced
- 1/4 cup kalamata olives, halved
- 1/4 cup fresh parsley, chopped
- 2 Tbsp olive oil
- 1 Tbsp lemon juice
- 1 tsp dried dill
- Salt and pepper to taste

Directions:

1. In a large bowl, combine chopped cauliflower, cherry tomatoes, cucumber, red onion, kalamata olives, and parsley
2. In a small bowl, whisk together olive oil, lemon juice, dill, salt, and pepper
3. Pour the dressing over the salad and toss to combine thoroughly

Tips:

- Chill in the refrigerator for 10 minutes before serving to enhance the flavors
- Consider adding grilled chicken or fish on top for a protein-rich meal

Nutritional Values: Calories: 120, Fat: 9g, Carbs: 10g, Protein: 2g, Sugar: 5g, Sodium: 170 mg, Potassium: 400 mg, Cholesterol: 0 mg

Lamb Koftas with Tzatziki Sauce

Preparation Time: 25 min

Cooking Time: 10 min

Mode of Cooking: Grilling

Servings: 4

Ingredients:

- 1 lb ground lamb
- 1/4 cup onions, finely chopped
- 2 cloves garlic, minced
- 2 Tbsp fresh mint, chopped
- 1 tsp cumin
- 1 tsp smoked paprika
- Salt and pepper to taste
- For the Tzatziki Sauce: 1 cup grated cucumber, squeezed dry
- 1 cup coconut cream
- 1 Tbsp lemon juice
- 2 Tbsp fresh dill, chopped
- 1 clove garlic, minced
- Salt to taste

Directions:

1. Mix ground lamb, onions, garlic, mint, cumin, paprika, salt, and pepper together in a bowl
2. Shape the mixture into small oblong shapes and thread onto skewers
3. Grill over medium heat for 10 minutes, turning occasionally
4. For the Tzatziki Sauce: combine cucumber, coconut cream, lemon juice, dill, garlic, and salt in a bowl and mix well

Tips:

- Serve koftas with a generous dollop of Tzatziki sauce
- Garnish with extra mint leaves for a refreshing touch

Nutritional Values: Calories: 290, Fat: 25g, Carbs: 3g, Protein: 14g, Sugar: 1g, Sodium: 220 mg, Potassium: 350 mg, Cholesterol: 80 mg

Roasted Eggplant with Tahini Dressing

Preparation Time: 10 min

Cooking Time: 40 min

Mode of Cooking: Roasting

Servings: 4

Ingredients:

- 2 large eggplants, sliced into 1/2 inch rounds
- 4 Tbsp olive oil
- Salt and pepper to taste
- For the Tahini Dressing: 1/4 cup tahini
- 2 Tbsp lemon juice
- 1 Tbsp water
- 1 clove garlic, minced
- Salt to taste

Directions:

1. Preheat oven to 400°F (200°C)
2. Arrange eggplant slices on a baking sheet and brush both sides with olive oil and sprinkle with salt and pepper
3. Roast in the oven for 40 minutes, flipping halfway through
4. For the Tahini Dressing: whisk together tahini, lemon juice, water, garlic, and salt until smooth

Tips:

- Drizzle the tahini dressing over the roasted eggplant before serving
- Sprinkle with parsley or pomegranate seeds for a touch of freshness and color

Nutritional Values: Calories: 210, Fat: 18g, Carbs: 12g, Protein: 3g, Sugar: 6g, Sodium: 120 mg, Potassium: 450 mg, Cholesterol: 0 mg

MEDITERRANEAN BAKED SEA BASS

Preparation Time: 15 min
Cooking Time: 30 min
Mode of Cooking: Baking
Servings: 4

Ingredients:

- 4 sea bass fillets, about 6 oz. each
- 2 Tbsp extra virgin olive oil
- 1 Tbsp fresh lemon juice
- 3 cloves garlic, minced
- 1 tsp dried oregano
- 1 tsp dried basil
- 1/2 tsp sea salt
- 1/4 tsp cracked black pepper
- 1 lemon, thinly sliced
- 1/4 cup kalamata olives, pitted and halved
- 2 Tbsp capers

Directions:

1. Preheat oven to 400°F (200°C)
2. In a small bowl, mix olive oil, lemon juice, garlic, oregano, basil, salt, and pepper
3. Place sea bass fillets in a baking dish and pour marinade over them, ensuring each fillet is well coated
4. Top fillets with lemon slices, olives, and capers
5. Bake in preheated oven for 25-30 min, or until fish flakes easily with a fork

Tips:

- Add fresh parsley and a drizzle of olive oil before serving for extra flavor and presentation
- Pair with a side of steamed asparagus for a complete meal

Nutritional Values: Calories: 280, Fat: 15g, Carbs: 3g, Protein: 34g, Sugar: 1g, Sodium: 620 mg, Potassium: 780 mg, Cholesterol: 85 mg

HARISSA-ROASTED VEGETABLES

Preparation Time: 10 min
Cooking Time: 40 min
Mode of Cooking: Roasting
Servings: 4

Ingredients:

- 1 lb. mixed vegetables (carrots, zucchini, bell peppers), chopped
- 2 Tbsp olive oil
- 3 Tbsp harissa paste
- 1 tsp cumin seeds
- 1/2 tsp sea salt
- 1/4 tsp black pepper
- 2 Tbsp fresh cilantro, chopped

Directions:

1. Preheat oven to 425°F (220°C)

2. In a large bowl, combine olive oil, harissa paste, cumin seeds, salt, and pepper

3. Toss chopped vegetables in the spice mixture until well coated

4. Spread vegetables evenly on a baking sheet

5. Roast in the oven for 35-40 min, stirring halfway through, until vegetables are tender and caramelized

Tips:

● Sprinkle with fresh cilantro just before serving for a burst of freshness

● Serve alongside quinoa or roasted chicken for a hearty meal

Nutritional Values: Calories: 200, Fat: 9g, Carbs: 28g, Protein: 5g, Sugar: 8g, Sodium: 300 mg, Potassium: 850 mg, Cholesterol: 0 mg

• 12.3 LATIN AND ASIAN FLAVORS

CHILEAN SEA BASS WITH MANGO SALSA

Preparation Time: 20 min

Cooking Time: 15 min

Mode of Cooking: Grilling

Servings: 4

Ingredients:

● 4 Chilean sea bass fillets (6 oz. each)

● 2 ripe mangos, peeled and diced

● 1 red bell pepper, finely chopped

● 1 small red onion, finely chopped

● ¼ cup fresh cilantro, chopped

● Juice of 2 limes

● 1 Tbsp olive oil

● Salt and black pepper to taste

Directions:

1. Preheat grill to medium-high heat (about 400°F or 204°C)

2. Season the fish fillets with salt and pepper and brush lightly with olive oil

3. Place fish on the grill and cook for about 7 min on each side or until cooked through

4. In a medium bowl, combine mango, red bell pepper, red onion, cilantro, and lime juice to make the salsa

5. Season the salsa with salt and pepper to taste

6. Serve the grilled fish topped with mango salsa

Tips:

● Serve immediately for the best flavor and texture

● Consider adding a dash of chili flakes to the salsa for a spicy kick

● Pair this dish with a side of grilled vegetables for a complete meal

Nutritional Values: Calories: 340, Fat: 12g, Carbs: 18g, Protein: 35g, Sugar: 13g, Sodium: 75 mg, Potassium: 950 mg, Cholesterol: 85 mg

KOREAN BULGOGI LETTUCE WRAPS

Preparation Time: 15 min

Cooking Time: 10 min

Mode of Cooking: Pan Frying

Servings: 4

Ingredients:

● 1 lb. lean beef, thinly sliced

● 2 Tbsp coconut aminos

● 1 Tbsp sesame oil

● 2 garlic cloves, minced

● 1 tsp fresh ginger, grated

● 1 Tbsp apple cider vinegar

● Salt and black pepper to taste

● 1 head butter lettuce, leaves separated

● 1 carrot, julienned

● 1 cucumber, thinly sliced

● Fresh cilantro for garnish

Directions:

1. Combine beef, coconut aminos, sesame oil, garlic, ginger, and vinegar in a bowl and let marinate for 10 min

2. Heat a skillet over medium-high heat

3. Cook the beef in the skillet until browned and cooked through, about 8 min

4. Assemble the wraps by placing some beef, carrot, cucumber, and cilantro in each lettuce leaf

5. Roll up the lettuce leaves to enclose the fillings

Tips:

● Use water chestnuts for a crunchy texture in the wraps

● Serve with a side of kimchi for authentic Korean flavor

● This dish is best enjoyed fresh due to the crispness of the lettuce

Nutritional Values: Calories: 200, Fat: 9g, Carbs: 6g, Protein: 26g, Sugar: 2g, Sodium: 320 mg, Potassium: 500 mg, Cholesterol: 50 mg

THAI COCONUT CURRY SHRIMP

Preparation Time: 10 min

Cooking Time: 10 min

Mode of Cooking: Simmering

Servings: 4

Ingredients:

● 1 lb. shrimp, peeled and deveined

● 1 can (14 oz.) coconut milk

● 1 Tbsp red curry paste

● 1 Tbsp fish sauce

● 1 tsp honey

● 1 red bell pepper, sliced

● 1 cup snap peas

● 1 small bunch basil, leaves torn

● 1 Tbsp coconut oil

● Salt to taste

Directions:

1. Heat coconut oil in a large skillet over medium heat

2. Add red curry paste and stir for 1 min

3. Pour in coconut milk, fish sauce, and honey and bring to a simmer

4. Add red bell pepper and snap peas and cook for 5 min

5. Add shrimp and cook until they are pink and opaque, about 5 min

6. Stir in basil leaves and season with salt

Tips:

● Serve with cauliflower rice for a low-carb meal option

● Garnish with additional basil leaves for enhanced flavor and presentation

● Adjust the amount of curry paste to tailor the heat level to your liking

Nutritional Values: Calories: 295, Fat: 18g, Carbs: 8g, Protein: 25g, Sugar: 3g, Sodium: 900 mg, Potassium: 460 mg, Cholesterol: 150 mg

ARGENTINIAN CHIMICHURRI STEAK

Preparation Time: 10 min

Cooking Time: 6 min

Mode of Cooking: Grilling

Servings: 4

Ingredients:

● 4 (6 oz.) sirloin steaks

● 1 cup fresh parsley, finely chopped

● 4 garlic cloves, minced

● 2 Tbsp red wine vinegar

● ⅓ cup olive oil

● 1 tsp dried oregano

● ½ tsp chili flakes

● Salt and black pepper to taste

Directions:

1. Preheat grill to high heat (about 450°F or 232°C)

2. Season steaks with salt and pepper ♪ Grill steaks for about 3 min on each side for medium-rare

3. Combine parsley, garlic, red wine vinegar, olive oil, oregano, and chili flakes in a bowl to make chimichurri sauce

4. Spoon chimichurri sauce over grilled steaks before serving

Tips:

- Let steaks rest for a few minutes after grilling to retain juices
- The chimichurri sauce can be made ahead and stored in the refrigerator to enhance its flavors
- Pair this steak with a fresh salad or grilled vegetables for a balanced meal

Nutritional Values: Calories: 410, Fat: 30g, Carbs: 2g, Protein: 32g, Sugar: 0g, Sodium: 65 mg, Potassium: 550 mg, Cholesterol: 90 mg

THAI BASIL GROUND BEEF STIR-FRY

Preparation Time: 10 min

Cooking Time: 15 min

Mode of Cooking: Stovetop

Servings: 4

Ingredients:

- 1 lb. ground beef
- 1 cup fresh Thai basil leaves
- 2 cups broccoli florets
- 1 red bell pepper, sliced
- 1 onion, thinly sliced
- 3 cloves garlic, minced
- 2 Tbsp coconut aminos
- 1 Tbsp fish sauce
- 1 tsp freshly ground black pepper
- 2 Tbsp coconut oil

Directions:

1. Heat coconut oil in a large skillet over medium heat
2. Add garlic and onion, sauté until translucent
3. Increase heat to high, add ground beef, breaking it apart, cook until browned
4. Add broccoli and bell pepper, stir-fry until vegetables are tender-crisp
5. Stir in coconut aminos, fish sauce, and black pepper
6. Just before removing from heat, add Thai basil leaves, stir until wilted

Tips:

- Serve immediately for best flavor and texture
- Can substitute Thai basil with regular basil if unavailable but flavor will differ
- Great with a side of cauliflower rice for a complete meal

Nutritional Values: Calories: 240, Fat: 15g, Carbs: 8g, Protein: 20g, Sugar: 3g, Sodium: 650 mg, Potassium: 350 mg, Cholesterol: 80 mg

CHAPTER 13: MAINTAINING A WHOLE FOOD LIFESTYLE

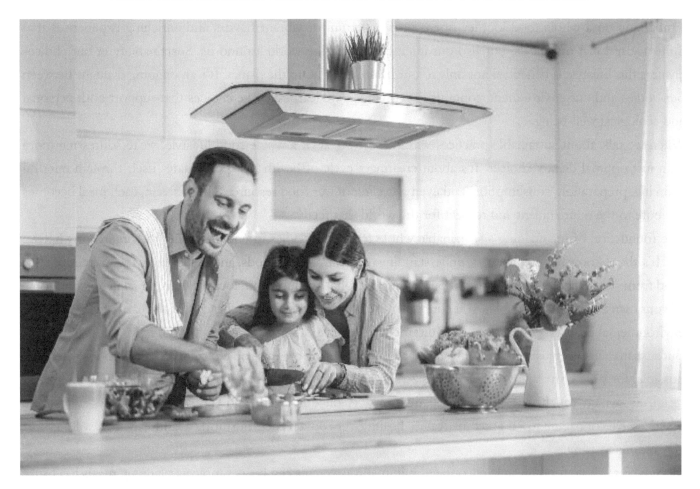

Embarking on a journey toward a healthier lifestyle through whole foods is a vibrant beginning, but the true magic lies in nurturing this practice into a sustainable part of your daily life. Imagine this: after thirty days of wholesome eating, you've started to notice the delightful changes—more energy, clearer skin, perhaps even a trimmer waistline. Yet, the real challenge often begins when the initial excitement wears off. How do you maintain this enriching whole food lifestyle amid the pull of old habits and the rush of everyday demands?

This chapter is your guide to transforming the 30-day challenge into a lifelong love affair with whole foods. Think of it as nurturing a garden. It starts with the joyous labor of planting—infusing your life with new, nourishing habits—and evolves into the ongoing, gentle gardening—tending and savoring the delicious fruits of your efforts. Like any seasoned gardener will tell you, the key to a thriving garden is consistent care and the occasional adaptation to changing seasons.

We will explore strategies that help embed these whole food principles deeply into your everyday routines. You'll learn how to listen to your body's signals, adapt recipes to suit fluctuating tastes and needs, and make conscious choices that prioritize your health and palate. More importantly, it's about crafting a joyful, food-filled life that feels as natural and refreshing as a home-cooked meal shared with loved ones.

Let's embrace the concept of mindful eating—not just as a diet but as a celebration of food that nourishes not only our bodies but also our souls. Through conscious choices, a sprinkle of creativity, and a dash of love, a whole food lifestyle is not just an occasional challenge; it becomes a rewarding, lasting way of life.

Embarking on a whole food journey opens up a spectrum of vibrant flavors and enriching experiences that influence not just our meals, but also our interaction with the world around us. Sustainability in our choices ensures this lifestyle is beneficial not only to our health but also to the planet. It's an ongoing dialogue between our bodies and our environment, continually evolving as we learn to make choices that support both personal and ecological well-being.

When we talk about sustainable practices within the context of a whole food lifestyle, we're addressing more than just optimal dietary choices. It's about creating a cycle of health that perpetuates itself through mindful sourcing, preparation, consumption, and even recycling of our food resources. In this vein, each meal becomes a tribute to the nourishment and respect for the world that feeds us.

The foundation of maintaining a sustainable whole food lifestyle lies in understanding the origins of what we eat. It's about knowing your farmers, understanding their farming methods, and recognizing the journey of your food from seed to table. When you start purchasing seasonal produce from local farmers, or even growing some of your own herbs and vegetables, you connect more deeply with the natural cycles of the earth and reduce the environmental costs associated with long-distance food transportation.

But sustainability isn't just about locality; it's also about choosing organic and ethically produced foods whenever possible. Organic farming practices emphasize soil preservation and avoid the use of synthetic pesticides and fertilizers, which can have long-term negative impacts on our health and the planet. By supporting these practices, we contribute to a market that values health over convenience, nurturing a landscape that will support generations to come.

Moreover, a whole food lifestyle encourages minimal waste. This can be as simple as planning meals to ensure all ingredients are used within the week, preserving foods to extend their freshness, or transforming leftovers into new, flavorful dishes. Composting organic waste further closes the loop, turning potential trash into nutrient-rich soil that can help grow more food. The act of composting not only reduces the trash that ends up in landfills but also connects us back to the earth, reminding us of the natural cycle that sustains us.

Sustainability extends into how we store and cook our foods. Investing in high-quality, durable kitchen tools and containers reduces the need for frequent replacements. Cooking methods also play a crucial role; using techniques like steaming or slow cooking can enhance food's nutritional value and taste while saving energy compared to higher-impact methods like frying.

Education is a pivotal component of sustainable practices. By educating ourselves and our families about where food comes from, how it's grown, and the impact our choices have on our health and the planet, we empower ourselves to make informed decisions. This isn't about making perfect choices all the time but about making better choices more often. It's also about spreading that knowledge—sharing sustainable practices with friends, participating in community gardens, or even advocating for food policy changes that support sustainable agriculture.

Engaging in a community of like-minded individuals can foster this lifestyle profoundly. Being part of a whole food community, whether online or in person, provides a reservoir of shared knowledge, motivation, and support. It's about building a network that celebrates whole, unprocessed foods and sustainable living, learning from each other, and growing together.

Maintaining a whole food lifestyle sustainably requires a dynamic approach. It's about adapting to life's changes and continuing to make choices that align with these values. Sometimes, it might mean choosing a less ideal but more accessible option when circumstances demand. The key is maintaining a flexible mindset and making the best possible choice at each opportunity.

Finally, it's important to celebrate the journey. Each step towards a more sustainable whole food lifestyle is a victory, deserving recognition. Celebrating these small successes fosters the process joyful and fulfilling and sets a positive example for others to follow. Remember, sustainability is a journey, not a destination. It is about moving forward, making conscious choices, and enjoying the bounty of health and harmony offered by a lifestyle that respects our bodies and our planet.

Thus, by weaving these practices into the fabric of daily life, sustainability becomes not just a concept, but a lived experience. It's an enriching path that enhances not only our own lives but contributes to a global heritage of health and ecological balance.

• 13.2 MINDFUL EATING

In the bustling rhythm of modern lives, our meals often resemble pit stops—quick refueling breaks amidst the chase of deadlines and commitments. However, adopting a whole food lifestyle is more rewarding when coupled with the practice of mindful eating—a technique that transforms these quick stops into moments of real nourishment, tranquility, and joy.

Mindful eating invites us to be fully present during our meals. It's a form of meditation at the table, where every bite is savored, and every flavor is appreciated. This practice not only enhances the sensory experience of eating but also fosters a deeper connection to our food, how it nourishes us, and acknowledges the effort that brought it to our plate.

The Essence of Mindful Eating

The core philosophy of mindful eating revolves around consciousness—being aware of the physical and emotional sensations associated with eating. This begins with choosing to consume whole foods that are healthful and sustaining, continuing to the way these foods are prepared, and finally, being truly present as we eat them.

Creating a Mindful Kitchen

The environment in which we prepare and consume our food can significantly influence our ability to eat mindfully. A cluttered, chaotic kitchen can subconsciously mirror a disordered approach to eating. In contrast, a clear and organized kitchen invites calmness, making it easier to engage fully with the preparation and consumption of food. Setting the stage for a mindful meal might involve clearing the dining space of distractions such as electronic devices or stressful paperwork, perhaps lighting a candle or playing soft music, anything that signals to the senses that this time is different, this time is for nourishment.

Engaging the Senses

Mindful eating teaches us to engage all of our senses in the act of eating. Notice the color, texture, and aroma before taking a bite. By appreciating these elements, we begin to tune into the natural cues our body gives about hunger and satisfaction which can lead to better portion control and a greater understanding of our body's nutritional needs.

Mindful Preparation

Cooking can be a meditative practice. Each step, from chopping vegetables to stirring a pot, can be done with mindful awareness. By focusing on these tasks, we ground ourselves in the moment, pushing away worries about the past or future, leading to a more serene state of mind that carries over to the eating experience.

Listening to the Body

Mindful eating involves listening intently to our body's hunger and fullness signals. It encourages eating slowly, which not only aids digestion but also gives the body time to signal when it has had enough. This helps prevent overeating and makes the act of eating an intentional practice rather than an automatic reaction.

The Emotional Dimensions of Eating

Food is not just physical nourishment but also comfort, celebration, and sometimes a coping mechanism for stress or sadness. Mindful eating encourages recognition and respect for these emotional dimensions without allowing them to dictate our eating habits. It helps distinguish between emotional hunger and physical hunger, guiding us towards better choices.

Mindful Eating in Everyday Life

Incorporating mindful eating into daily life doesn't require perfection. Start by choosing one meal per day to eat mindfully or setting a weekly date where dinner involves all the aspects of mindfulness. As with any habit, the more it's practiced, the more natural it becomes.

Challenges to Mindful Eating

Distractions are one of the biggest challenges to eating mindfully. In a world where multitasking is often celebrated, choosing to do just one thing—eating—can feel unproductive. However, this single-task focus allows for a richer, more connected eating experience and ultimately, a more healthful relationship with food.

Long-term Benefits of Mindful Eating

Adopting mindful eating doesn't just change the way we eat—it changes the way we live. Over time, it fosters a greater appreciation for the little things, a calmer approach to life's challenges, and a healthier, more balanced relationship with food. It can lead to lasting weight management, improved digestion, and decreased stress eating, profoundly impacting overall wellness.

In embracing the techniques of mindful eating, we embrace a lifestyle that honors our food and ourselves. It teaches us to slow down, to savor the moment, and to recognize the incredible journey food takes to reach our plates. More importantly, it reminds us that each meal is a reflection of our respect for our body, our health, and our world.

• 13.3 ONGOING SUPPORT

Embarking on a whole food journey is akin to setting sail on a vast, vibrant ocean. The initial thrust into the waters of change is exhilarating, filled with the excitement of new flavors and the pride of healthy choices. However, as with any continuous voyage, the challenge often lies in maintaining momentum amidst the routine waves and occasional storms. Ongoing support is the compass that helps navigate these waters, ensuring that the journey towards health and wellness is not only begun but continued and cherished.

Understanding the Need for Support

Let's begin by acknowledging a fundamental truth: change, especially when it involves lifestyle habits, can be challenging. The initial days are often bright with novelty but maintaining the course requires more than just initial enthusiasm. This is where ongoing support plays a crucial role – it acts not just as a safety net, but as an active catalyst that fosters long-term success and enjoyment in the whole food approach.

Types of Ongoing Support

Community Connections: Often underestimated, the power of community is profound. Engaging with like-minded individuals who are also embracing whole food lifestyles provides motivation and encourages accountability. Local support groups, online forums, and social media platforms can connect you to whole food enthusiasts around the world. These relationships empower sharing of tips, recipes, and encouragement, making the journey less solitary and more communal.

Professional Guidance: Occasionally, you might seek advice that goes beyond the conversational support of peers. Nutritionists, dietitians, and even culinary experts specialized in whole foods can offer professional insights tailored to your specific health needs and culinary tastes. These professionals not only help in structuring dietary plans that align with your health goals but can also assist in overcoming specific nutritional challenges.

Educational Resources: Knowledge is a powerful tool in maintaining any lifestyle change. Books, documentaries, workshops, and cooking classes dedicated to whole foods and healthful living can enhance your understanding and appreciation of your dietary choices, reinforcing your commitment. Keeping abreast of the latest research in nutrition also helps refine your approach as new findings emerge.

Digital Tools and Apps: In this digital age, technology offers immediate support right at your fingertips. From apps that help track nutrient intake and grocery planning to those offering whole food recipes and meal ideas, the digital world is equipped to support your dietary habits robustly and innovatively.

Regular Health Check-ups: Another aspect of ongoing support involves monitoring your health through regular check-ups. These not only track progress but also preemptively address potential health issues. Understanding the impact of a whole food diet on your body through professional medical advice is invaluable.

Integrating Support in Daily Life

Integrating support effectively requires recognizing its importance in your daily routine. This might mean scheduling weekly meal planning, setting regular intervals for community meet-ups, or allotting time each month to explore new educational materials. The idea is to create a support system that is both robust and flexible, capable of adapting to your changing lifestyle and needs.

Emotional and Psychological Support

The journey toward maintaining a whole food lifestyle isn't just physical. It's deeply emotional and psychological. Support groups or counseling services can provide the space to discuss struggles and triumphs not just in dietary terms but in how these changes affect your emotional world. Understanding and managing the emotional responses to dietary change is crucial in maintaining a balanced approach to whole food living.

Celebrating Milestones

Incorporating celebration into this support framework is essential. Celebrate milestones big and small with your community, family, or support team. These celebrations reinforce positive outcomes and provide motivation. Whether it's mastering a new whole food recipe or hitting a health milestone, each deserves recognition and serves as a reminder of the progress made.

Lifelong Learning and Adaptation

Finally, ongoing support for a whole food lifestyle means embracing the idea of lifelong learning and adaptation. As life evolves—age, health changes, lifestyle adjustments—so too might your dietary needs. Support systems must be dynamic, capable of adapting to these changes to provide relevant and effective guidance.

In conclusion, ongoing support is a multifaceted and dynamic aspect of maintaining a whole food lifestyle. It encompasses personal connections, professional advice, educational growth, and emotional counseling—each element playing a vital role in nurturing and sustaining your dietary choices. This tailored support ensures that your journey is not just about food but about cultivating a fulfilling and health-conscious lifestyle. Through this network of support, the whole food lifestyle transforms from a mere dietary choice into a joyous, life-enhancing journey.

Made in United States
Troutdale, OR
04/05/2025